MAKE EVERY BREATH COUNT

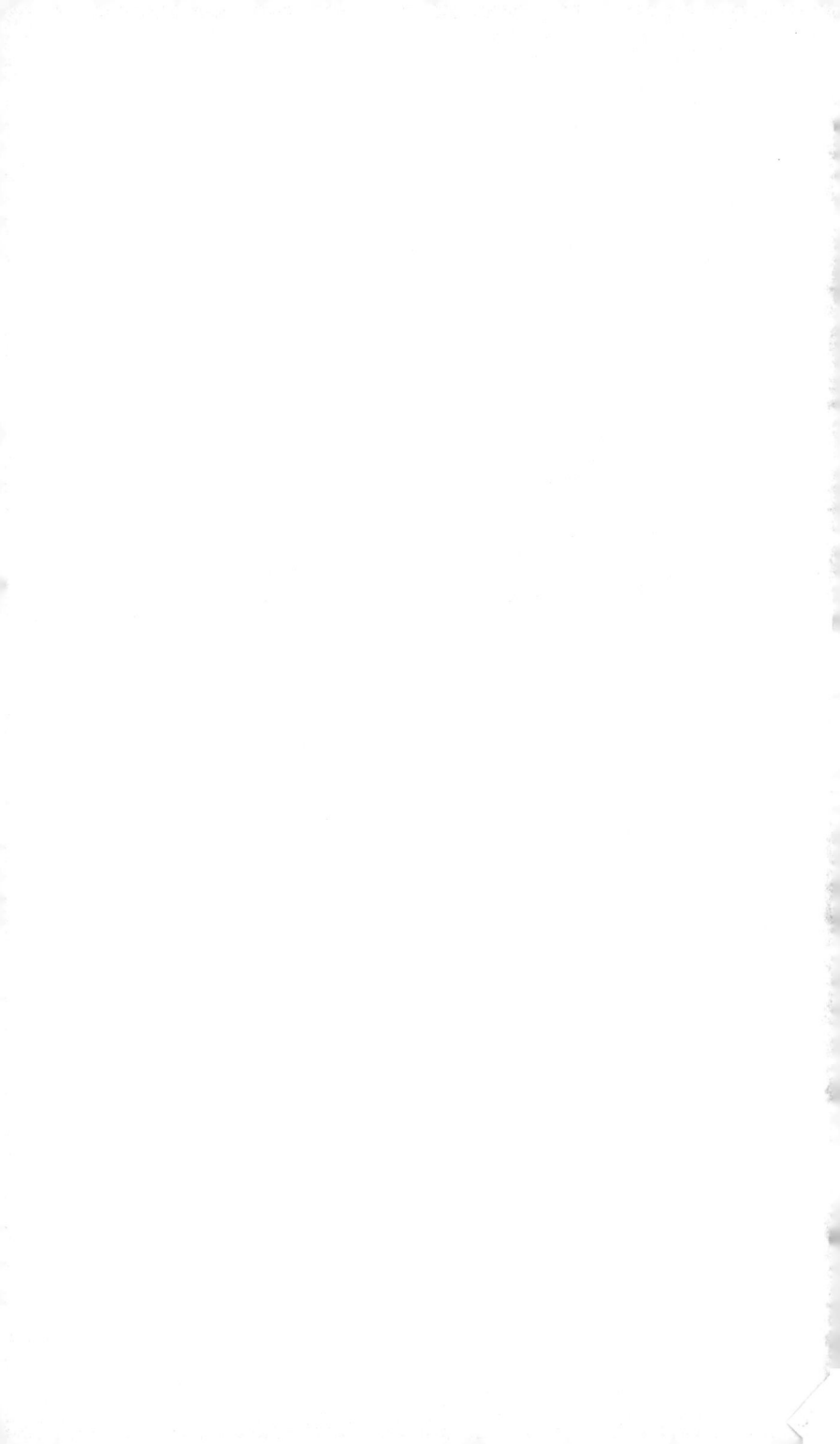

MAKE EVERY BREATH COUNT

Science And Stories Of The
Lung-A Pulmonologist's Narrative

———————

Dr Pallavi Periwal

Copyright © 2023 by Pallavi Periwal

Illustrations copyright © 2023 by Pallavi Periwal

All rights reserved. No part of this book may be reproduced, stored in a retrieval system or transmitted, in any form or by any means, without the prior written consent of the publisher

Cover design by Ritika Periwal

The advice provided in this book has been carefully considered and checked by the author. *The content of this book is for informational purposes only and is not intended to diagnose, treat, cure, or prevent any condition or disease. You understand that this book is not intended as a substitute for consultation with a licensed practitioner. Please consult with your own physician or healthcare specialist regarding the suggestions and recommendations made in this book. The use of this book implies your acceptance of this disclaimer.* You also understand and acknowledge that you should never disregard or delay seeking medical advice relating to treatment or standard of care because of information contained in or transmitted through this book.

Medical information changes constantly. Therefore the information in this book should not be considered current, complete or exhaustive, nor should you rely on such information to recommend a course of treatment for you or any other individual.

Neither the author nor the publisher or their representatives shall bear any liability whatsoever for personal injury, property damage, and financial losses.

To my parents,
For raising me to believe that
anything is possible

Contents

Acknowledgements 1

Preface 3

About the Book 6

PART ONE: MAKING SENSE OF LUNGS: KNOWING HOW IT WORKS 9

Respiratory System: A closer look 11

Inhale Exhale: Mechanics of the Machinery 18

PART TWO: MYTHS, REALITY, AND PREVENTION 25

Lung Cleanse: How Do I Keep My Lungs Healthy? 27

Early Predictors of Lung Disease:
Navigating Early Symptoms and Risk Factors 43

You Are What You Breathe 57

Sleep and Lung Health: The Surprising Connection 69

Clearing the Air: Dispelling Myths Around Lung Diseases 76

PART THREE: BEYOND THE PANDEMIC 83

The COVID-19 Pandemic: Reflections and Lessons 85

The Aftermath: Post Covid-19 Syndrome 90

About the Author 97

Notes 98

Acknowledgements

Writing a book is much harder than I had imagined it to be. Here I take a moment to express my heartfelt gratitude to those who have offered me profound support in my writing journey. I would not be here if it were not for them.

First, my baby boy, Samar, I thank you for bringing so much happiness into my life. Your cheerful presence and ability to find joy in little things have been a constant reminder to appreciate the simple pleasures in life.

Second, I would like to thank my husband, Ruchir, for being with me through thick and thin. The person who made me start this book and the one whose encouragement and eye-rolls have led to its completion. Thank you for always being there with a listening ear and hot coffee.

I am thankful to my father, Tarun, for teaching me hard work . I appreciate your unwavering support, your willingness to read my drafts, and your constructive feedback. Thank you for making me feel safe to do big things in the world.

Again, I am thankful to my mother, Shalini, for believing in me more than I ever believed in myself. For always being encouraging and positive. Thank you for feeding me love and hot delicious food always.

My sister, Ritika, I am grateful for making my illustrations look beautiful and the book cover spectacular. Thank you for always being there to make me laugh, to challenge me, and to remind me that I am not, in fact, the centre of the universe (even though I like to think otherwise).

I am grateful to my teacher and mentor, Dr Deepak Talwar, for teaching me pulmonology like no one else could and for instilling the love of the subject in me. I also thank Dr Arjun Khanna for being a guide and friend and for being my go-to person for all the difficult questions I have.

Also, I thank my friends for always looking out for me and helping me be my best.

Finally, I am thankful to my patients who shared their stories, their struggles, and their laughter with me. Thank you for teaching me resilience and empathy.

Preface

It all started with Covid.
In August 2020, I was diagnosed with COVID-19 pneumonitis. Well, I diagnosed myself. Fortunately, I wasn't sick enough to be hospitalized, or so I like to think. Maybe I set the level of sickness requiring hospitalization too high for myself. Why, you might ask. I was scared. Just like anyone else in the world, maybe a little bit more because I knew to some extent the havoc the virus was causing, seeing these patients every day.

You see, I am a pulmonologist. A rare speciality, that not many people knew about in the pre-COVID era. I deal with patients who have respiratory diseases, diseases that affect the lungs. So I constantly see individuals with breathing difficulties and coughing bouts in my practice. I also see people with allergies and sleep problems. I also treat patients who are admitted to the Intensive Care Unit (ICU) because of respiratory issues. Therefore, I have experienced a considerable number of patients dealing with lung problems.

When COVID broke, there was no proper treatment guideline available, and the norms for isolation were strict, really strict. I went on to be isolated for 21 days. That was the time when the community spread of the virus had just started in India.

Everyone knew someone who had COVID-19. It was the time most people got to know that a lung specialist is called a pulmonologist. The media were calling us to seek a better understanding of the disease. Everyone wanted an answer. "How scary is this virus? Will it get worse? Will vaccines help?" These were some of the pertinent questions they asked. To be quite frank, no one knew all the answers at this time; research had already started on a lot of aspects related to COVID-19. Numerous papers related to the disease were published in various journals. So much so that it was hard to keep up with them; I am sure my colleagues would agree.

At this time, few researchers had started researching the lungs and ways to keep them healthy. Also, advice and precautionary measures were shared on WhatsApp and other social media platforms to help people remain safe.

During this time, myths related to the disease were spreading fast. Really, I cannot count the number of times people asked me if drinking *kadha* would kill the virus. *Someone should create awareness,* I thought.

COVID spread rampantly all over the country, making frontline health workers extremely busy and exhausted. I began to write blogs on topics that I felt needed to be addressed. These were only a handful, not because there was little to be discussed or little misinformation spread among people, but because I was always short on time.

In the last three years, the pandemic has taught all of us lessons—lessons about work, about health, and about people. For me, these have been both personal and professional. It seems interesting to me that a tiny virus has the potential to change our perspective on life itself.

For many people, the pandemic has been life-altering, and some of the horrid moments are starting to fade from our memories now. I don't want to refresh those memories because it was a tense time. No one wants to relive those days, so we will not dwell on those stories. So what is this book about? What can a pulmonologist have to say that might interest you?

About the Book

Tell me if this sounds familiar. You got diagnosed with COVID-19. You were really unwell for some days. You promised yourself you would take better care of your condition. So you started some self-care and healthy practices during the lockdown. Eventually, you recovered and felt better once more. The lockdown got over, COVID cases reduced drastically, you went back to working full time at your office, and you got back to the same habits you had before the pandemic. Now, every few weeks, the media reports about the number of cases rising in China and the United States of America. A new variant of the virus is discovered somewhere else in the world, potentially virulent, but no one knows for sure what is going to happen, and you are reminded of the habits you wish you had continued.

Well, you are not alone. We tend to forget things when the harm perceived reduces.

Wouldn't it be wonderful to know and live a lifestyle that keeps your lungs and overall health in good shape?

This book is for anyone who has had COVID-19 or any other respiratory disease. Also, it is meant for anyone who wants to give their children a healthy start and anyone who has a family member with a respiratory illness. Additionally, it is meant for those desirous of understanding how the lungs work and improving their lung health. When your baseline lung is in an optimum function, and you have good immunity, you tend to recover better and faster. This book is not about COVID-19. It is a book about the lessons from the stories and science of the lung. I have tried to keep it short and to the point, cutting away all the fluff but with stories from my practice to make it interesting and impactful. I have changed the names and identifying characteristics of all patients to protect their identity.

The way to read this book is simple. Read it from the first page to the last. Do not skip to portions that you feel are interesting; you will skip important information if you do so. It is not a long read, and the writing style is easy to read. I keep in mind that most people who will read this have no working knowledge of medicine. If you have an average reading speed, you should be able to finish the book in two hours. That, I would say, is a short time to gain some insight into your lungs.

To begin with, we will take a closer look at the mechanics of the lungs and how they work to keep us breathing. We will then explore different ways to cleanse and support your lungs, including exercises and lifestyle changes.

Further into the book, I will tell you seemingly simple objects—which you think pose no harm—that might actually harm your lungs. We will also discuss the relationship between sleep and lung health. Toward the end, I debunk some myths about lungs and clear some misconceptions surrounding respiratory diseases. Finally, in the last section, we will discuss how to take care of post-COVID lungs and cover lessons we can learn from the pandemic about life in general.

Whether you're a curious student, a health-conscious individual, or a medical professional, this book is packed with profound information to help you improve your lung health. I hope you find it informative and engaging and that it serves as a valuable resource in your quest for better lung health.

Happy reading!

For anyone wondering: Drinking *kadha* does not kill the virus. *(Kadha is a drink made with a number of herbs and spices that are boiled in water to extract their benefits.)*

(PART ONE)

MAKING SENSE OF LUNGS: KNOWING HOW IT WORKS

Respiratory System: A closer look

September 2004

"Maybe we should skip lunch," I said.

"Why is that?" my friend asked.

"I just don't think it is such a brilliant idea to eat," I replied

"You are being paranoid," my friend said.

"Am I?"

"Come on, it's just lunch. Nothing will happen."

"No, you go ahead, I will skip lunch," I decided, and so I did.

This was my second month as a medical student, and we were going to have our first dissection class that day. For those of you who don't know what that means, a dissection class is a practical anatomy session where you have to see dead bodies preserved in formalin (or cadavers as there are called in the science community) and study the human anatomy on them. Back in those days, YouTube had not even started, so we had to rely on books and bodies.

We entered the dissection hall with our noses scrunched up, making weird faces. The smell in the room was horrible; it was the smell of preserved human bodies. Interestingly, it was scheduled after lunch. Why did they arrange the anatomy practical class right after we ate? Well, maybe I was thinking too much. I thought the smell in the anatomy lab from the formalin would make me vomit. That did not happen, thankfully.

As much as I had thought I would detest it, I quite enjoyed dissection. Weird, you might think. But actually, we were taught to think of cadavers as our resources. A sea of knowledge. This was the first time that I actually saw and touched human lungs. We cut down a part to identify the various structures inside. I will never forget the feeling of holding human organs in my hands. It felt surreal.

Normal human lungs weigh about 1-1.3 kg combined and are light pink in colour. That's right, pink. But as we go through life, aging and inhaling toxic air, they turn black. Here we will find out about what our lungs look like and how they develop as we grow up.

When we breathe, the air travels through our nose into the pharynx to the windpipe (trachea) into the lungs. The human body has two lungs or a pair of lungs: right and left lung. Now both the right and the left lung have the same function in our body, but they are not identical. There are more like siblings than twins. Why they are different is not important, but why they are essential to us is.

Our lungs lie in our chest cavity, secured by the ribcage on all sides and muscles, fat, and skin on top. They are almost conical in shape, the apex of which points upwards. The heart lies between our two lungs. And together, the three rest on top of a thick muscle, separating them from the abdomen. This is called the diaphragm.

Each lung is divided into smaller areas called lobes. The right lung is divided into three lobes, while the left is divided into two. The thing that divides them is called a fissure, so the right side has two fissures, and the left has one. Both the lungs are covered by an extremely thin membrane called the pleura (Pronounced as PLU-RA)

The windpipe, upon reaching the lungs, divides into two parts called the left and right bronchus. And as they travel further into the lungs, they divide further like the branches of a tree. After 20-22 of such divisions, the hollow tubes form alveoli (AL-VEO-LI) or air sacs.

Once air reaches the air sacs, it comes in contact with blood vessels inside the lungs for the exchange of gases. Oxygen is delivered to the lungs, and carbon dioxide is taken back into the air sacks and then up the hollow tubes into the trachea, and finally out through the nose. The alveoli are extremely tiny; they are invisible to the naked eye, and yet they are powerful. They make gas exchange possible and provide oxygen to the entire body.

The complex cycle of breathing, which occurs around 20,000 times a day, occurs mostly without us knowing about it. It is automatic, and it occurs at a subconscious level.

We don't realize how many things we do subconsciously. You woke up today, brushed your teeth, got ready, and drove to work, all the while not thinking specifically about those things. Rather you thought about other things while doing them. Like, *I hope there is no traffic today. Did I email that presentation? Did I make the credit card payment?* Similarly, we are used to not being aware of our breathing. It is not a job for us. It is something our body does for us, and so we tend to take it for granted.

LUNGS

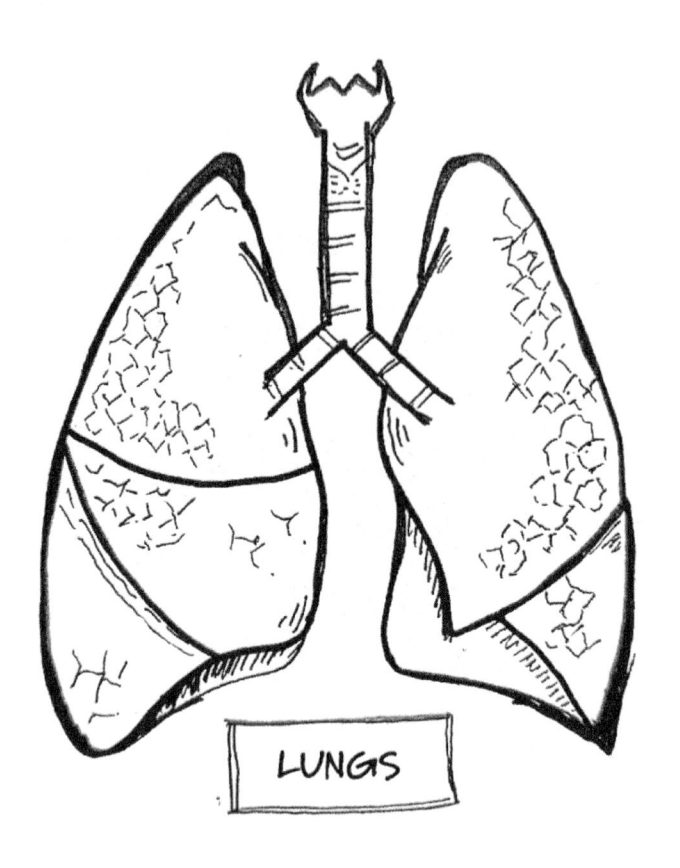

Tracheobronchial Tree

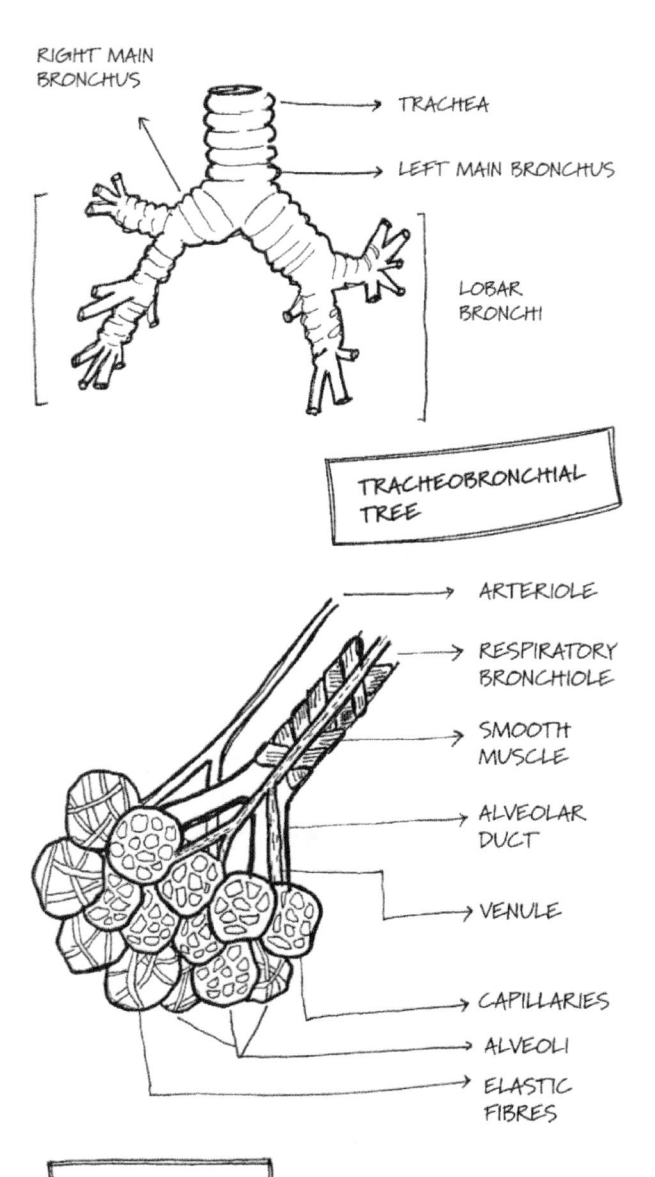

- RIGHT MAIN BRONCHUS
- TRACHEA
- LEFT MAIN BRONCHUS
- LOBAR BRONCHI

Alveoli

- ARTERIOLE
- RESPIRATORY BRONCHIOLE
- SMOOTH MUSCLE
- ALVEOLAR DUCT
- VENULE
- CAPILLARIES
- ALVEOLI
- ELASTIC FIBRES

November 2004

I was holding my embryology book in hand and thinking, *why did I decide to become a doctor?* Embryology is the study of embryos or the life within the mother's uterus. It is one of the most difficult topics I have had to deal with. How does one imagine something they have never seen, and then to make matters even more complicated, how do you imagine its parts and how it develops?

The journey of a human embryo is so complicated that when a baby is born normal, it has already fought a great deal in its embryo life to come this far. They have dodged numerous developmental abnormalities before coming to the world.

The development of the lung is nothing ordinary too. When the human embryo is as old as four weeks, the development of the respiratory system starts, and by 36 weeks, the entire system is formed. But our lungs continue to form new air sacs until 20 years of age.[1]

The cells that make up our lungs are tiny, yet they perform one of the most powerful functions in the body. The closest thing that humans have made, which works as an alveoli, is a ventilator. The ventilator is so much larger. Do you marvel at the human body?

August 2007

As a third-year medical student, my life was about learning to take patient histories and examining them. This is the time medical students flaunt their stethoscopes around their necks, and we began to get a sense of what being a doctor will feel like.

But the first time you use the stethoscope to listen to a patient's chest, you feel lost.

"Can you hear anything? Can you hear a bronchial breath sound?" my senior resident doctor asked.

I should be able to hear something, I thought. The patient looked at me, annoyed, as this was the tenth time I had asked him to take a deep breath in and then exhale. I smiled nervously at him. Surely, I should be able to hear it. Everyone in my clinical group had. At the cost of not sounding stupid, I said, "Yes, I can hear it".

"Good, pass on the stethoscope to the next student," he said, rather irritated.

And so, I did. This batchmate of mine did not hear anything either. I could see it in his eyes. I felt a sense of relief. Thank God I was not the only one.

When we breathe in and out, the passage of air through the hollow tubes (Trachea and bronchi) produces sounds. These are called lung sounds, which can be heard using a stethoscope. These sounds change if the lungs are unhealthy or diseased. Breathing is the most important function of the respiratory system, but it is not the only one.

Inhale Exhale:
Mechanics of the Machinery

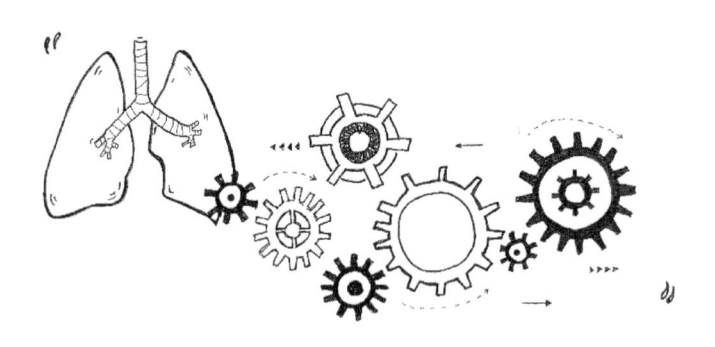

There are several hundred million alveoli in our body, and the combined surface area is estimated to be 70m^2, which is half the size of a tennis court.[1] That is enormous. Imagine how complex the human body is to be able to fit that inside our lungs.

July 2004

Just a few more days to go before I started my life as a medical student. August 1 was going to be the D-day—the day that changed my life to make it what it is. Now, I don't know if getting into any under-graduation program requires you to get a medical check-up, but the journey of becoming a doctor starts with that. I had just given my blood samples and gotten a chest X-ray done. I was reluctantly waiting for the X-ray report in the waiting area with my mother.

"Here you are," said the peon.

"Thanks," I hurriedly took the brown envelope from him, took the X-ray out, and tried to figure out what I could possibly see.

Of course, I did not understand anything. So I quickly put it back.

"That's the way all doctors look at X-rays," said a man, sitting behind me in the waiting area, smiling.

He was my batchmate's father, a doctor himself. I smiled back hesitatingly. What a foolish person he must think I am. Trying to read X-rays before even starting medical college.

Ever since then, I have been fascinated by X-rays. A film with only shades of grey and black. Yet, it can tell you what is wrong with the lungs, whether a person is being able to breathe normally or not, and to tell if they have pneumonia or lung cancer. It was much later in my training that I was able to understand X-rays properly.

Breathing comprises of inhaling (taking the air in) and exhaling (slowly releasing air out). When we inhale, our diaphragm muscle contracts, flattening and moving downward, creating more space in our chest cavity. At the same time, our intercostal (rib) muscles contract, pushing the ribcage up and out, further increasing the space in the chest cavity. The increased space in the chest cavity creates a negative pressure, which draws air into the lungs through the nose or mouth, down the trachea, and into the bronchial tubes.

Once the air reaches the bronchial tubes, it branches out into smaller tubes called bronchioles. At the end of each bronchiole are clusters of tiny air sacs called alveoli. These alveoli have extremely thin walls, allowing oxygen to diffuse easily into the bloodstream while carbon dioxide diffuses from the bloodstream into the alveoli. The oxygen-rich blood then travels to the heart, where it is pumped to the rest of the body to provide energy to the cells. Meanwhile, the carbon dioxide-rich blood returns to the lungs, where it will be exhaled during the next step of the breathing cycle.

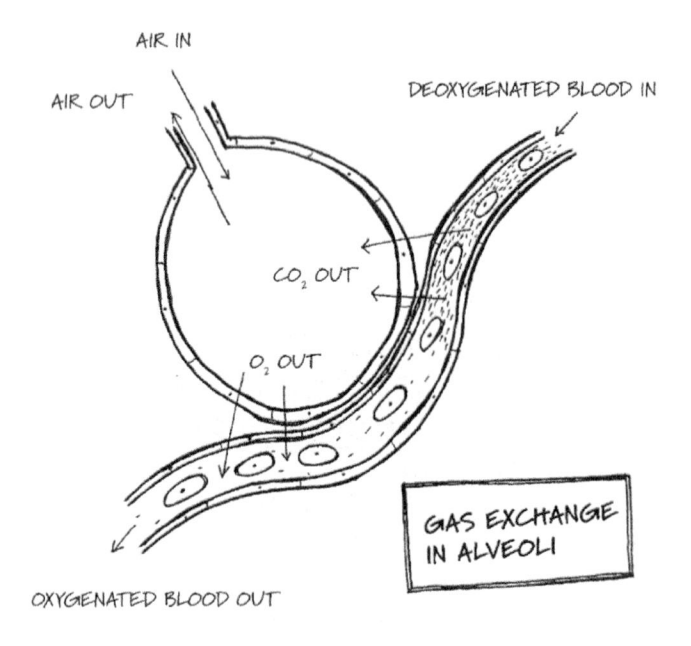

AIR IN

AIR OUT

DEOXYGENATED BLOOD IN

CO_2 OUT

O_2 OUT

GAS EXCHANGE IN ALVEOLI

OXYGENATED BLOOD OUT

When we exhale, the diaphragm muscle relaxes and moves back to its original position, and the rib muscles relax, causing the ribcage to move back down. This decrease in space in the chest cavity increases the pressure in the lungs, making it easier to push the air out. The air travels back up the bronchial tubes, through the trachea, and out of the nose or mouth. This cycle carries on, keeping us alive.

It's important to note that breathing is not just a passive process, but rather it is regulated by our respiratory system, which includes the lungs, trachea, bronchi, bronchioles, alveoli, and the muscles that control breathing (diaphragm and intercostal muscles). This system works together to ensure we get the oxygen we need and remove the carbon dioxide waste.

The respiratory system starts at the nose and ends at the alveoli. When we inhale, our nose takes in the air and filters it before sending it further down. All dust particles and bacteria of a certain size are filtered out by the nose. The nose also helps with the function of smell.

The lungs do not only help us breathe; they also have many critical functions in the body. We call these the non-respiratory functions. The lungs also help in speech production. The passage of air in hollow tubes produces sound, and by providing the necessary airflow for speech sounds, the lungs, and vocal cords work together to make it possible for us to speak, sing, or even shout.

Additionally, the lungs protect our heart by acting as shock absorbers surrounding it. Along with the kidneys, they maintain our body's pH balance. They protect us against infections and foreign invaders by producing immunity-boosting IgA antibodies. The tiny hair-like structures called cilia in our bronchial tubes move in coordinated, sweeping motions to clear out mucus and other particles, preventing them from reaching our lungs.

Moreover, the lungs help in non-verbal communication. Breathing patterns and the sounds of breathing can provide nonverbal cues about our emotional state, level of exertion, or illness. For example, rapid and shallow breathing can indicate anxiety or fear, while heavy breathing can indicate physical exertion.

The lungs are closely related to the heart. They are like cousins who live in the same house. The heart is the youngest, always protected by the lungs on both sides. The heart is dependent on the lungs to provide it with oxygenated blood and remove all the impurities from the blood. Much like a younger sibling is dependent on the older one to show them the way and keep toxic things away from them. The heart and the lungs are connected by pulmonary blood vessels. Any changes in one of the two would lead to changes in the other via this connection.

March 2010

Finally, I am a doctor. MBBS is done with. What a relief!

I was excited and also a little scared because I knew it didn't stop there. Now I had to do post-graduation. My subject of interest was Medicine. You get to see a bit of everything, all kinds of patients. After a quick discussion with my friend's older sister, who was a doctor, I decided I was going to take USMLE (US Medical Licensing Examination) and do my residency in internal medicine in USA. That was the plan.

Now USMLE is a tough nut. It has three parts, and the whole process is pretty lengthy. I got to it, got excellent scores, and now I was set to apply to colleges for interviews. I applied. Unfortunate circumstances did not lead to a Match. Now a match is when you basically get assigned a university. I was shocked. *How is that possible? I have excellent scores, I have letters of recommendation, I have experience as an observer in the USA. My interviews went really well. Is there a problem with the computer algorithm that did not select me?* I thought to myself. I was almost in denial.

I had always been a good student. So when I wasn't admitted, I felt devastated. At least, at that point, it was. After two years of relentless studies, this was heartbreaking. I spent my days in my room, locked up so no one would disturb me. I read for 12-14 hours a day and only came out for meals. My mother would just see me at meal times. I didn't attend family functions or go to weddings or get-togethers. All this for nothing. *This is not fair. Life is not fair,* I thought.

Meanwhile, some of my friends got through to good universities in the USA. "Maybe you should try again next year", they encouraged.

"Ya, maybe," I said. But my heart wasn't in it anymore. It was too much of a disappointment for me. You might think I just quit at that point. But really, I decided to reroute. *Maybe this is just not the way for me. Maybe I have to try something else. Maybe there is some meaning to it.* I thought. I began preparing for Indian post-graduation exams.

I had already missed the dates for all Indian postgraduate exams and some other entrance examinations since I was in the USA at that time. So the next exam was DNB (Diplomate of national board).

December 2012

I got through the DNB entrance exams. The counselling session to decide on the specialty that I was going to was to occur soon. Every day I sat in front of my computer to see the remaining subjects. General medicine seats were vanishing like hotcakes. This was not going to be easy to get.

By the time it was my chance, only respiratory medicine seats were left. *This seems close enough to medicine. At least I will get to use my stethoscope.* That was my only consolation. I wasn't completely happy with it, but I did not have a choice. It was either this or waiting for another six months for another exam, and frankly, I had had enough. I was sick of taking exams.

Specialization in respiratory medicine, that's what it is going to be.

(PART TWO)

MYTHS, REALITY, AND PREVENTION

Lung Cleanse: How Do I Keep My Lungs Healthy?

May 2013

My first month as a junior resident was extremely stressful—well, actually, the first six months. But the first month was exceptionally so. I had a 36-hour shift and had an inadequate sleep. I did not eat well and did not understand much on the rounds or in the classes, and felt extremely tired. All junior residents went through this, and I was no exception. My life was all about the hospital and the patients.

Things were much calmer on Sundays. The Consultant round was relaxed. There was no rush to finish tasks, there were no classes, and there was a general atmosphere of calmness. So on a particular Sunday morning, I had some free time and went to chat with one of the patients. She was a 65-year-old lady who had been asthmatic all her life. But this was the first time she was admitted. She did not understand why. I explained that she had pneumonia, an infection that affects the lungs, and so it required admission. She asked me, "Is there a way to protect my lungs? How can I stay healthy?"

Over the years, many patients have asked me, "What are the ways to keep my lungs healthy? How can I ensure my lungs are fine? How can I take care of my lungs?" Some people already have lung diseases, some have no problems, and more recently, they have either suffered from or are afraid of being infected by COVID.

My answers to these questions lead to another question. What do you do to keep your body healthy? The answer is a bit obvious now—anything that keeps your body healthy, keeps your lungs fit and in good shape. But there are definitely a few extra things that you can do to ensure you suffer from lesser respiratory issues.

As we grow older, so do our lungs. Our bones, including the ribs, get weaker and thinner, muscles lose their strength, the air sacs become less efficient in gas exchange, and the lungs become more prone to develop inflammation and infections. Our body's ability to fight foreign particles and germs decreases. Therefore, if we stop taking good care of our body or our lungs, we will have a difficult old age.

This chapter discusses what you can do to keep your lungs in good shape. These are simple, practical things that you can implement to help your heart realize its optimum function.

Know your BMI

Rather than being obsessed about your weight, calculate your Basal Metabolic Index (BMI). (BMI= Weight (Kg)/Height^2 (Metres)). Your BMI is a better measure of your weight than your height. Although it doesn't take into account factors such as age, gender, ethnicity, and the physical activity of a person.

For an average Indian, the normal BMI is 18.5-23 Kg/mt^2. If your BMI is less than 18.5Kg/mt^2 you are underweight, and if it is over 23 Kg/mt^2 you are overweight. If it is greater than 25 Kg/mt^2 you are obese.[1]

These values vary among ethnicities, and the World Health Organization (WHO) has a different classification. However, according to the Indian guidelines, any Indian with BMI greater than 25 Kg/mt^2 is obese and stands the risk of getting diabetes and heart diseases.

If you are overweight, it will affect your breathing mechanism. Accumulation of fat in the chest and abdominal cavity can impede the inflation of the lungs. This results in poor lung function, which translates into breathing difficulties. It has been found that people who are obese have to breathe more often, have to exert more effort to overcome the resistance of the airways, and are more often hypoxic (have lower oxygen levels in blood).

Common lung diseases associated with obesity include Asthma, Obstructive Sleep Apnea (OSA), and Obesity Hypoventilation Syndrome (OHS). Obesity causes systemic inflammation and increased oxidative stress, which may induce asthma in obese patients. The risk of developing asthma is increased by 1.5–2.5 folds in overweight people, and the risk of being hospitalized is 4–6-fold higher for obese asthma patients. In obese asthma patients, exacerbations are more frequent, and asthma is less under control while the quality of life is reduced. 'Obese asthma' is a separate phenotype or category which scientists believe is more difficult to treat, as response to medications is poorer.

OSA is a disease where the upper airway collapses during sleep and leads to obstruction in the flow of air to our lungs, thus briefly stopping breathing. Obesity causes the collapse of upper airways through fat accumulation in the face, neck, and pharynx. We will be discussing this further in the book.

OHS is a condition where morbidly obese patients have poor breathing, which leads to reduced oxygen levels and increased carbon dioxide levels in the blood. The mechanism of this disease is complex, but to oversimply it, an increase in the fat tissue around the lungs, on the muscles, chest wall, and diaphragm, along with a blunted response from the brain centre makes it extremely difficult for the person to breathe effectively.

Studies have shown that a weight loss of >5% of the initial weight can improve the symptoms of Asthma and OSA; however, for significant improvement in OHS, a patient needs to lose up to 25-30% of the body weight.[2]

Being underweight or malnourished is not a good sign either. It will make you more susceptible to infections with viruses, bacteria, and other organisms.

Healthy Eating Habits

We all know the importance of healthy eating habits, yet it is something we often take for granted. People often are aware that certain foods can cause gastrointestinal trouble, heart problems, or even sometimes cancer. However, I have never come across anyone who thinks that food is closely related to the lungs. Our body works on two fuels: food and oxygen. Food is changed into energy, and this process is called metabolism. The right mix of nutrients is required to make breathing easy. To make things easy, remember to include all five food groups in your diet on an everyday basis. These are carbohydrates, proteins, oil and fats, fruits and vegetables, and dairy products.

Carbohydrates should form the base meal for the body. They are essential because they provide the body with the energy to carry out breathing and other tasks. These include food like wheat, brown rice, kidney beans (rajma), chickpeas, lentils, jowar, bajra, corn, beetroot, potato, sweet potato, oats, banana, apple, mango, raisins, dates, etc. Where possible use the wholegrain variety; they are rich in fibre and starch and keep you full for a long time.

Food rich in protein to be included are lentils, eggs, fish, chicken, meat, milk, oats, cheese or panner, almonds, peanuts, and pumpkin seeds. They help the body to grow and repair itself. It is essential to eat lean cuts of meat and skinless poultry, as they contain lower fat. Limit the intake of red meat. Protein helps to keep your muscles strong, including your chest muscles, which help your ribs expand as you breathe. This helps you get the most out of exercise and pulmonary rehabilitation (PR). It is also important for your immune system.

Good oil and fat should be included in small quantities as they are an important source of essential fatty acids. They help absorb Vitamins A, D, and E. A good diet should include more unsaturated fats than saturated or trans fats. There is good evidence that replacing saturated fats with unsaturated fats can help to lower your cholesterol level.

Food rich in saturated fats includes butter, ghee, cream, biscuits, cakes, palm oil and coconut oil, and fatty cuts of meats. Trans fats are found in partially hydrogenated vegetable oil. Adults should not consume more than about 5g of trans fats a day. These include deep-fried food, packaged baked food, and processed packaged food.

Unsaturated fats are of two types: monounsaturated fats (MUFA) and polyunsaturated fats (PUFA). These help lower the level of bad cholesterol in the body. MUFA is found in olive oil, rapeseed oil, avocados, and some nuts, such as almonds and peanuts. PUFA includes omega-3. Omega-6 fats cannot be made by your body, which means it's essential to include small amounts of them in your diet. Omega-6 fats are found in vegetable oils, like rapeseed, corn, and sunflower oil, while Omega-

3 fats are found in oily fish. Other sources of Omega 3 fats are flaxseed oil, rapeseed oil, soya oil, tofu, and walnuts.

Good amounts of fruits and vegetables should be included in the diet. These provide fibre, vitamins, and minerals. Eat five portions of fruits and vegetables a day. Each portion is about 80gm of fruit or vegetable or 30gm of dried fruit. Make it easy to remember by including a variety of colours in your diet. These will help build your immunity.

Milk and dairy products are good sources of protein and calcium. It is especially important to include calcium in your diet if you are taking steroids for your medical conditions to prevent bone loss or osteoporosis. A common misconception is that certain dairy products cause cough or phlegm. However, there is actually no substantial research to prove that milk or other dairy products cause these conditions. Unless you are allergic or lactose intolerant, it is alright to consume them. If you feel that it causes mucus to thicken or makes it difficult to expectorate, just drink some water or rinse your mouth following it.

Another very pertinent question I am asked is if nutritional supplements are required. All essential vitamins and minerals are provided if you consume a well-balanced diet. In case of any deficiencies, these supplements may be added. In certain patients with chronic illnesses, it is best to consult the doctor before taking supplements.

Antioxidants in the lung are the first line of defence against oxygen-free radicals. Non-enzymatic antioxidants, such as vitamin C (ascorbic acid), vitamin E (alpha tocopherol), and b-carotene, a precursor of vitamin A, ubiquinone, flavonoids, and selenium, are present in foods. These influence several components of our immunity.

There is no concrete evidence supporting the role of multivitamins and supplement pills in boosting your immunity.

Further long-term studies, mainly randomizing patients into two groups, where one is given the supplement and the other a placebo, would be required to establish the impact of nutrient intake on the occurrence and progression of the disease and to determine optimal doses.

It is also essential to drink enough water to keep your body hydrated. A good measure of hydration would be to see the colour of your urine. Darker urine suggests inadequate water intake. The quantity of water varies depending on each person.

August 2013

I was sitting in the doctor's office, completing a patient's file. He was 50 years old and had come in with the acute onset of breathing difficulty. After an initial treatment with medicines, he started to feel better. It was almost lunchtime now. From the corner of my eye, I saw this patient reach out for his lunch and start to eat. In less than 5 minutes' time, he was breathless again. Then the nurse and other staff ran to his aid. I join them.

This is a common scenario in a respiratory ward. Oftentimes, the patient is unable to eat properly when he/she is breathless. The following are some rules to aid eating when you suffer from a lung condition that causes breathlessness:

- Eat slowly: Chew your food properly and take small bites of food.
- Eat soft and moist food in contrast to hard and difficult to swallow food.
- Try to sip water while you eat to facilitate the swallowing of the food.
- Avoid food that causes bloating.
- If you feel you cannot eat solid food, try semi-solid or liquid form for a few days and then switch back to solids when you are more comfortable.
- Split your meals into 4-6 smaller meals.

- Do not overeat.
- If you are very uncomfortable eating, avoid eating altogether. Let your doctor know. They will let you know an alternate arrangement.
- Avoid lying down while eating or drinking; it increases the risk of aspirating and causing inflammation in the lungs.

Exercise

Exercise can have a significant impact on lung function and respiratory health. Any physical activity counts as exercise, including sports ike running, swimming, tennis, or hobbies such as cycling or walking, and daily activities like walking to the shops.

For good health, aim for 30 minutes of moderate exercise at least five days a week. Brisk walking at 4-6 km/h is suitable for healthy individuals, while those with lung problems should aim at a pace causing moderate breathlessness.

Regular exercise can improve lung function by increasing the strength and capacity of the respiratory muscles. As a result, the lungs are better able to deliver oxygen to the body during physical activity. This is especially important for athletes or individuals who engage in endurance sports such as running, cycling or swimming.

In addition to improving lung function, exercise can also have a positive impact on lung health by reducing the risk of respiratory diseases such as asthma, chronic obstructive pulmonary disease (COPD) and lung cancer. Regular exercise has been shown to strengthen the immune system, which can help protect against respiratory infections.

However, it is important to note that certain types of exercise can also have a negative impact on lung health. High-intensity exercise, particularly in environments with poor air quality, can lead to an increase in respiratory symptoms such as coughing, wheezing, and shortness of breath. This is especially true for individuals with pre-existing respiratory conditions such as asthma or COPD. If you suffer from exercise induced asthma, it is important to take your bronchodilator 10 minutes before you exercise to prevent exercise-induced bronchoconstriction.

It is important for individuals with respiratory conditions to consult with a healthcare professional before starting an exercise program. This will help ensure that the exercise program is safe and appropriate for their specific needs.

The importance of breathing technique cannot be underestimated. Breathing through the nose, rather than the mouth, can help filter out pollutants and allergens in the air, improving lung health. It is also important to maintain a steady breathing rhythm during exercise to ensure that the body is receiving adequate oxygen.

It is important to incorporate both aerobic and strength-training exercises into an exercise program. Aerobic exercise, such as running or cycling, can improve lung function and cardiovascular health, while strength-training exercises can help strengthen the respiratory muscles.

The following are essential tips to keep in mind during exercise for a safe and effective workout:

- Warm up: Start with gentle activities involving the muscles you will use during your workout. This helps to prepare your body for the more intense exercise ahead.
- Stretch: Improving flexibility through stretching exercises can help prevent injury and improve performance.

- Build stamina: Gradually increase your ability to exercise for longer periods, allowing your body to adapt to the demands of your workout.
- Increase activity at your own pace: It's important to push yourself, but don't be afraid to get slightly out of breath. A good rule of thumb is to aim for a 4-5 on a scale of 0-10 for intensity.
- Improve muscle strength: Incorporating strength-training exercises, such as weight lifting, can help improve overall fitness and prevent injury.
- Cool down: At the end of your workout, gradually slow down your activity and stretch the muscles you've used. This allows your body to gradually return to its resting state and helps prevent injury.

By following these tips, you can help ensure a safe and effective workout, improving your overall fitness and helping you achieve your fitness goals.

Yoga

If you google the benefits of yoga, you will find numerous articles. In the last two years, I have come across many such write-ups and articles telling us about the benefits of yoga, especially for your lungs. The question, however, is, does yoga really help keep your lungs healthy? Is pranayama good for your lungs? If you are like me, then you like to research things before you believe them.

There is no doubt yoga is recommended for a number of conditions, from anxiety and depression to neurological conditions and cancers. However, existing studies have only been able to recommend yoga as an add-on therapy to support a person.

Yoga is a form of exercise that can have a positive effect on the lungs and respiratory system. Yoga practices such as pranayama (breathing exercises) and asanas (yoga postures) can help to improve lung function and capacity. Pranayama, specifically, can help to increase lung capacity and improve the efficiency of breathing. These exercises can help to strengthen the muscles used for breathing, increase the flexibility of the chest and diaphragm, and promote better oxygenation of the body.

Yoga can also have a positive impact on the mind-body connection and stress management, which can, in turn, have a positive impact on lung health. Practicing yoga regularly can also improve overall well-being and reduce the risk of lung-related diseases such as asthma and chronic obstructive pulmonary disease (COPD).

In 1999, Christopher Gilbert published a paper on yoga and breathing. He posits that "the body of knowledge, beliefs, and practices comprising yoga emphasizes control of breathing as central to its ideals and its goals. The fact that control of breathing is also central to most methods of relaxation, meditation, and body control indicates at least that it is popular, and it is probably popular because it works. Many of the claims for yoga have not been tested yet by current standards of science, and some of the variables are so intangible that testing seems futile. But physiological and medical research is confirming many of the claims based originally on observation and tradition."

The study also reveals that certain principles run through most of the exercises (in yoga) and are considered fundamental to good breathing, whatever the circumstances. These principles are:

- Abdominal breathing is better than chest breathing
- Breathing through the nose is preferable to breathing through the mouth

- Slow breathing without rushing the exhale is beneficial
- Smooth, steady breathing is preferable to irregular choppy breathing
- Observing one's breathing is good.

It's important to note that yoga should be performed under the guidance of a qualified yoga teacher, especially for people with lung or respiratory conditions. In my opinion, if your doctor says it is safe for you to practice these breathing exercises, you can go ahead with them.

Vaccines

Vaccines have been one of the most effective public health measures in preventing and controlling infectious diseases. Not only do they protect individuals, but they also help to prevent the spread of diseases within communities. Vaccines have been developed to prevent a wide range of infections, including lung infections caused by viruses and bacteria.

Vaccines work by stimulating the immune system to produce antibodies against specific infections. When a person is vaccinated, a weakened or dead version of the virus or bacteria is introduced into the body. This prompts the immune system to recognize the virus or bacteria and produce antibodies against it. If the person is later exposed to the actual virus or bacteria, their immune system is ready to recognize and fight it off, preventing the person from getting sick.

There are several vaccines that help protect against lung infections. These include:

Influenza vaccine: The flu vaccine is an annual vaccination that helps protect against influenza viruses. It is recommended for people who are at higher risk of complications from the flu, such as elderly people, pregnant women, and people with certain medical conditions.

Pneumococcal vaccines: Pneumococcal vaccines protect against pneumococcal bacteria, which can cause pneumonia, meningitis, and other serious infections.

The pneumococcal vaccine is available in two forms: the pneumococcal conjugate vaccine (PCV) and the pneumococcal polysaccharide vaccine (PPV). The PCV is typically given to infants and young children as part of the routine childhood vaccination schedule, while the PPV is recommended for adults over the age of 65 and for people with certain medical conditions that put them at higher risk of pneumococcal disease.

It is important to note that while the pneumococcal vaccine can provide protection against some strains of pneumococcal bacteria, it does not protect against all strains. Additionally, the vaccine does not protect against other common causes of pneumonia, such as viruses or other bacteria.

COVID-19 vaccine: The COVID-19 vaccines has been shown to be highly effective in preventing COVID-19, which can cause severe lung damage and respiratory failure.

Other vaccines that prevent against respiratory infections are pertusiss vaccine against whooping cough and BCG (Tuberculosis Vaccine) against disseminated tuberculosis (TB) and the more serious forms of TB like TB meningitis which affects the brain. Both these vaccines are given in childhood.

Lung infections can be serious and even life-threatening, especially for people who are at a higher risk, such as young children, the elderly, and people with weakened immune systems. Vaccines are one of the most effective ways to prevent these infections and protect vulnerable populations.

In addition to protecting individuals, vaccines also help prevent the spread of infections within communities. When enough people are vaccinated, it creates herd immunity, which means that the disease is less likely to spread, even among those who are not vaccinated. This is important because some people cannot receive certain vaccines, such as those with weakened immune systems, and rely on others to be vaccinated to protect them from infections.

Home environment- cleaning

October 2013

One week to go, and it would be Diwali, my favourite festival. Things were festive all around. Shops and buildings were lit all around. The markets were busy and chirpy. The most exciting part was that I was home this Diwali since I was not on duty that day. What a wonderful feeling! I was sitting in the intensive care unit, taking a break from seeing patients and daydreaming. The phone rang, and they were shifting a young patient with breathing difficulty from the emergency room.

Then I got a tap on my shoulder, "Dr Pallavi, the patient is here." Young patients with low oxygen levels are a scary preposition. This young man had breathing difficulty, which started around 10 am and quickly progressed to a level where he required high levels of oxygen at around 3:30 pm. It seemed very sudden. He had no prior records of having any respiratory illnesses. There was no family history of lung diseases. There was some improvement with treatment, but the most intriguing question was what had happened to him and why?

Once his breathing got a bit better and he was able to speak a few sentences, we asked him again about the sequence of events leading up to his symptoms. This time he told us he was cleaning his house for Diwali, and to clean his bathroom, he made a combination of bleach and hydrochloric acid mixture, and soon after, his symptoms started.

This young man had suffered from Reactive Airway Dysfunction Syndrome (RADS). A combination of these cleaning supplies can cause damage to the airways. Sometimes, it can precipitate an asthma attack, and this is not an unusual occurrence. This may be an extreme case. But a lot of people suffer from various extents of allergies and breathing issues because the day-to-day cleaning triggers it. Most of them are not aware of this trigger. Of course, one cannot abandon it altogether because if dust accumulates, it will cause more trouble for you. But one can work to minimize the exposure.

If you have a tendency to get sneezing or get watery eyes when cleaning, then it is important to take some safety measures. Use a cloth/ mask to cover your nose and mouth while cleaning. Don't mix chemicals, especially when working indoors. Keep the exhaust fans on when using chemicals. If someone else is cleaning, try to stay away from that area.

There are simple steps you can do to keep your lungs in optimum function. Probably you already know about a few of them. The focus here is to keep it simple and try to practice small things in our lifestyle, not just for healthy lungs but also for a healthy body and mind.

But what do you do if you have some respiratory symptoms? When do you consult a specialist? What special tests are needed and why? What are some red flag signs? In the next section, we will address these essential questions.

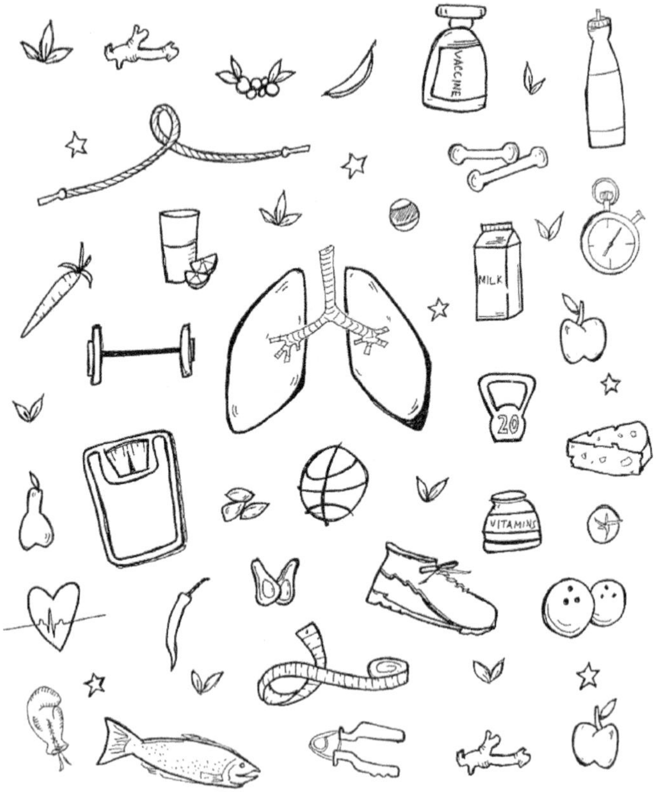
VACCINE
MILK
20
VITAMINS

Early Predictors of Lung Disease: Navigating Early Symptoms and Risk Factors

T he best thing that you can do for yourself is to not fall ill. However, often times that is not in our hands. In fact, most of the time, it is not up to us. You can take the best care of yourself and still suffer from a problem. So then, what is the next best thing to do?

The next most important thing to do is to recognise the symptoms you have as early as possible so that you can be diagnosed and treated early. More often than not, people miss these early signs and report to the doctor late, and sometimes the disease may have progressed to an irreversible stage.

Early Predictors of Lung Disease

I have treated hundreds of people with respiratory diseases and chronic illnesses of the lung in my professional practice. Some get better fast, some have a stable disease that remains as such for a long period in their lives, while others have illnesses that progress very fast, causing them to fall ill often. Apart from the fact that every disease has its own natural course, which means its progression and end state is well studied and known, there is one significant factor that determines whether you will recover from the illness or if the disease will progress fast, and that is how soon the problem is detected and how soon the treatment is started.

The sooner the symptoms are identified and dealt with, the better the outcome. This has been my general observation for not just diseases of the lung but other organs as well.

When you know what symptoms are worrisome and should be reported to a doctor, you empower yourself and give yourself the gift of early diagnosis. Not only can you start treatment early, but a lot of times, you can also nip the disease at its root.

There are some key symptoms that can predict lung diseases early on, and these are called the cardinal symptoms of the respiratory system. They are cough, breathing difficulty, sputum production, chest pain, wheezing (or noisy breathing), and blood in your cough. We will discuss them in detail shortly.

Often you may have a combination of these symptoms, like cough and breathing difficulty, or there can be one of these with another symptom, such as cough and weight loss. The important thing to remember is that if you experience any of the above six symptoms, pay attention to your condition.

It is particularly a matter of concern if you have risk factors. Now what are these risk factors? These are factors that can put you at risk of lung diseases. It would be nearly impossible for me to list all of them here, but I will name the most common risk factors. If you are or have been a smoker in the past, are exposed to fumes/dust/ smoke/ toxins (inhalational), have pets, or have been in contact with someone with an infectious disease like tuberculosis or COVID, take your symptoms a bit more seriously. Also, if you have a family member with a lung disease, you may have it too.

It is important to note that lung diseases do not only affect people with high-risk factors; however, those with risk factors are advised to be more cautious.

March 2014
A 64-year-old gentleman, Mr Kailash, walked into my OPD room with his son.

"Please take a seat," I said.

Mr Kailash sat on a stool next to me. I noticed that he was averagely built, but his clothes appeared a bit loose in him.

"So what brings you here," I asked.

"I had some blood in my cough this morning. Can you give me some medicine for it? I have to go to a wedding in three days. So, I just want to make sure it doesn't happen there," he explained.

"Let me ask you a few more things to find out what it could be and then…"

"It is nothing," he cut me short, "just happened once in the morning."

"Please answer a few questions for me. Without that, I can't give you any medicines," I said, and reluctantly he agreed.

I asked him details about the blood colour—if it was mixed with food and if he had ever had this episode before. But he denied anything unusual.

"Do you have a cough?"

"No."

His son jumped in, "He does have cough, especially in the morning. Some days it is more, some days less. He doesn't take any medicines for it."

"Do you have breathing difficulty or chest pain?" I asked.

"No, I haven't noticed". His son jumped in again, "He doesn't walk as much now, he used to go for regular walks, but now it says they tire him." This is often another way how patients describe difficulty in breathing: not being able to do activities that they previously did.

"Any weight loss?"

"Yes, maybe little, but that is because I am not eating well since my wife passed away last year."

"Oh, I am sorry".

"Do you smoke, Mr. Kailash?"

"No," he replied. "He used to smoke," said the son.

"But that was 20 years ago. I have left for so long now," Mr. Kailash retorted.

I finished my questions on smoking and other symptoms. I requested some blood tests and a chest X-ray and told them to come back to me with the reports.

"This is really not required. You are making a big deal out of it. And I don't even have so much time left before the wedding," he protested.

"Mr. Kailash, these are simple tests, and you can get them done today, and we can discuss the plan first thing tomorrow when the reports are available."

His son agreed and took his father for the tests.

The following morning, my first patient on the list was Mr. Kailash. The reports were already in the file. One look at the Chest X-ray almost confirmed my suspicion.

I called them in and showed them the X-ray and what appeared to be a large white patch on his right lung.

"It seems like there is a problem in the right lung. There are some possibilities, but we now need a CT scan of the chest to confirm it. If the CT scan suggests the possibility of cancer, we will have to biopsy it."

Mr. Kailash's son appeared worried. "Can this wait a few days?"

"I wouldn't suggest you to wait. The sooner you get it done, the better it will be."

In the next few days, the CT scan and biopsy confirmed his condition to be lung cancer. Further tests were done to stage the disease and know what line of treatment could be offered to the patient. Unfortunately, it had already spread to his liver, and there was only chemotherapy to offer.

Often, when a grim diagnosis such as cancer is given to a person, they feel guilty, as though if they had done something differently, they would have avoided it altogether. And that is true in the case of Mr. Kailash, who was an ex-smoker. Smoking increases your chances of getting lung cancer. But then, even non-smokers get lung cancer. It might be of a different kind requiring a different treatment. Therefore, what could have been different in this scenario is early detection. If symptoms are identified early, cancer can be detected at an early stage, where it may be treatable with surgery and have a good long-term outcome.

The guilt of knowing that you could have done something different to get a different outcome in life is unimaginable. No one should have to live with that. If we pay close attention to what the body is saying, if we identify new symptoms and don't attribute them to things that we think may be causing them, we might be able to diagnose diseases much earlier than we currently do.

Cough

....

Everybody will cough at some point in their life. But not all cough is considered abnormal. It is a protective reflex of the body. Cough helps removes dust, mucus, and germs away from the body. But at some point, cough is an indication of an underlying problem in the lungs, especially when it is associated with other symptoms. Cough can be triggered by your occupation, environmental issues, exposures, or travel.

When the cough is present for three weeks or less, it is called acute cough. In most cases, an acute cough is usually self-limiting. It will clear up on its own without requiring treatment. Sometimes it will need a short course of treatment and will resolve soon. It could be due to upper respiratory tract infections affecting the throat, windpipe, and sinuses like cold, flu, pharyngitis, laryngitis, sinusitis, or whopping cough. Lower respiratory tract infections such as acute bronchitis or pneumonia affecting the lungs and lower airways can also produce these symptoms. There can be various other causes, such as allergy, hay fever, dust or smoke inhalation, and exacerbation of underlying diseases like Asthma, COPD, etc.

Some studies have suggested that in children, honey can be used to provide some relief in bringing down the duration of cough if used for three days. However, honey should be avoided in infants less than one year of age, as they may get clostridium botulism.

When it lasts from three to eight weeks, it could be due to post-infectious or non-infectious reasons similar to either acute or chronic cough. When the cough lasts for more than eight weeks, it is called chronic cough.

This can be due to certain types of medication one is on, upper airway cough syndrome due to sinus diseases, asthma, gastro esophageal reflux disease, or non-eosinophilic asthmatic bronchitis.

Every person who has been diagnosed with cough will be asked about certain signs he/she may have that could be a potentially life-threatening cause of cough. Any associated blood in cough, weight loss, fever, hoarseness of voice, trouble swallowing, and significant smoking history are all important signs of taking urgent action.

Cough can be dry or productive, where one brings up phlegm. Your doctor will be able to tell you more about the underlying lung problem based on this.

Sputum

The mucus and debris that you bring up from your lower airways and lungs are called sputum (phlegm). Some amount of mucus production is normal by the body. But if the amount is in excess or causes disturbance in your day-to-day activities, it can be a cause of concern.

A change in colour of the sputum from whitish to yellowish or greenish indicates an infection. The texture or consistency of sputum may also change from watery and clear to a darker and thicker, somewhat pus-like consistency indicating an infection.

The best way to find out about the cause of sputum is usually a sputum examination along with a chest X-ray and other relevant tests.

Blood in Cough

Few people cough out blood, and this can be scary. Sometimes the sputum is just streaked with few specks of blood, and at other times it is just blood. The amount of blood will depend on the underlying cause of this bleeding and can sometimes be so intense that it will land the patient in the emergency department of the hospital.

Blood coming out of anywhere from the body is never a good sign. It is always good to report this to a doctor and get a proper checkup done.

The first thing your doctor will try to figure out is whether it is truly blood and if it is coming out of the lungs or if you are vomiting it due to a problem in your gastrointestinal system. They will ask you about the colour of blood, if it is red or brownish, whether there are any food particles mixed with it, and if there are any other associated symptoms.

You will need some tests to find out why this happened, and in most cases, the doctor will be able to tell you what the cause of it is. Sometimes though, things are not that straightforward, and you will require a battery of tests before a conclusion can be reached.

One of the commonest causes of blood in cough in our part of the world is tuberculosis. It is a benign treatable condition, and if diagnosed on time, the recovery rate is one hundred percent. Another common cause could be cancer. When diagnosed early, it can be treated and controlled, depending on the kind of cancer it is and the stage of the disease.

There are numerous other causes, and these include lung infections, clots in lung blood vessels (pulmonary embolism), or even auto-immune diseases which affect the lung.

The first instance of blood in cough should alert you and make you want to see a doctor.

Shortness of Breath

At some point in our lives, we all get short of breath. Is it always due to some disease? The answer is No. Then when is it that you should worry about being short of breath?

In medical language, shortness of breath is also called dyspnea. It is defined by the American thoracic society as "a subjective experience of breathing discomfort that consists of qualitatively distinct sensations that vary in intensity." A person may define it as an increased effort to breathe, chest tightness or pain, and 'air hunger'- the sensation of not getting enough air. It is important to evaluate it by assessing the intensity of sensations, the degree of distress, and the impact on the patient's daily activities.

This sensation of breathlessness can be crippling for most people. It may occur over a period of a few minutes to a few hours (Acute dyspnea), or it may occur over a period of certain years (Chronic dyspnea). Acute dyspnea is usually promptly dealt with by people because it is sudden and really discomforting. Chronic dyspnea is often ignored. There are numerous reasons people 'think' they get breathless, often ranging from 'Oh, I am getting old' to 'My mother had similar issues, I think it is hereditary.' You might be right; it could be something you inherited from your parents, but it could still be treatable. It could be because you are aging, but more often than not, there is some underlying problem that needs to be dealt with.

Often, patients, when asked directly if they feel breathless, will tell me they don't, but their tests would suggest otherwise. These people are poor perceivers.

There are many causes of breathlessness. Broadly speaking, these can be divided into three categories: lung problems, heart problems, deconditioning and misc. Lung problems include infections such as lung infections, chronic obstructive pulmonary disease (COPD), asthma, and interstitial lung disease, among others. Heart problems could include pulmonary edema and myocardial infarction (often referred to as a heart attack). Deconditioning following prolonged bed rest or physical inactivity and other miscellaneous causes include anxiety or panic attacks.

The presentation of breathing difficulty is different for different causes. That is, some diseases have an acute presentation, like a heart attack, while others are chronic, like asthma.

Oftentimes, breathing difficulty is accompanied by other respiratory symptoms such as wheezing or chest pain, or cough. In these situations, it is imperative that you get yourself checked.

Your doctor will recommend blood tests, X-rays, and often a pulmonary function test to diagnose the underlying problem.

Wheezing

Wheezing is a high-pitched sound produced by the narrowing of the airways. The narrowing of airways could be due to partial blockage as a result of mucus and other debris, or it could be due to spasms of the airways. The muscles have to work really hard against this to be able to breathe out and, in the process, produce this whistling sound.

If you observe wheezing, it is almost always a cause of concern and should be reported and investigated early enough. Most of the time, it is accompanied by other respiratory symptoms like breathlessness, cough, or chest pain.

The most common cause of wheezing is asthma, although there are many other causes too, like COPD, heart failure, bronchitis, hypersensitivity pneumonitis, and sometimes even lung cancer, or a foreign body stuck in one of the airways. Your doctor will try to figure out if the wheeze is coming from one or both sides of the chest to know what the cause may be. Specialized tests like an X-ray of the chest, Lung function tests, and sometimes even a specialized CT scan of the lungs will be required.

Sudden disappearance of the wheeze is a red flag sign as it could mean complete obstruction of the airways. If you observe a bluish discoloration of your fingertips, mouth, or skin (called cyanosis), you should immediately go to an emergency room.

Sometimes wheezing occurs after eating new food or medicine or a bee sting, this is most likely due to an allergic or anaphylactic reaction and will require urgent medical care in an emergency.

The definitive treatment for a wheeze is the treatment of the underlying cause. There are some things that can be done at home. First, if you are a smoker, now is the time to stop smoking. Cut down all or any exposure to smoke. Practice deep breathing exercises. Use an air purifier with a HEPA filter. Use a humidifier or a vaporizer to moisten the air that you breathe to help relax the airways. It is also essential to consume warm fluids.

Chest pain

Usually, the first reaction to chest pain is, 'Am I getting a heart attack?' The pain of a heart attack (or myocardial infarction as it is called in medical terms) is usually on the left side of the chest, sometimes the centre. It may radiate to the left arm or back. It occurs for a few minutes or may come and go. It usually feels as if someone is constricting the chest and putting pressure on it. Along with this, there is breathing difficulty.

Agreed that a heart attack seems frightening, but not all chest pains are equal to a heart attack.

Chest pain can be due to a number of reasons. It can happen if there are problems with the lung, heart, gastrointestinal system, or muscles over the chest. Conditions of the lung include pneumonia, COVID-19, pleurisy, asthma, pulmonary embolism, or pulmonary hypertension (both involving the vessels connecting the heart and lung). Heart problems include heart attack or Myocardial infarction and problems with heart valves or lining. It also includes gastric issues like reflux and indigestion or pancreatitis. Muscle strain or spasm, inflammation of the rib cartilage (costochondritis), skin infection over the area overlying the chest, like herpes, and even pain attacks can cause chest pain.

The nature of chest pain varies for these conditions, and often, pain is accompanied by other symptoms. Chest pain due to reflux often comes with nausea and vomiting. Chest pain due to pneumonia is associated with cough and fever. This is a differentiating point for knowing the underlying cause for a doctor. But many times, these conditions may mimic each other and can be difficult to distinguish just based on the history of a patient. It is important to first rule out life-threatening conditions, and for this, tests are required.

Most often, these symptoms occur in different combinations for different diseases. Some require urgent attention, while for some others, you may observe over a period of time and then consult a doctor.

Here are some red flags to be checked out by a pulmonologist without delay if you have never had any prior respiratory illness:

1. Blood in sputum
2. Cough of more than two weeks duration
3. Breathing difficulty that is progressively increasing
4. Acute onset breathing difficulty in a previously healthy person
5. Chest tightness and associated wheezing
6. Unexplained weight loss in a smoker

In my professional practice, I have seen people give a number of reasons for not getting checked by a doctor. Some reasons are legit, while others are just excuses. I have had patients come in late with blood in their sputum because they did not think it was possible for them to have lung cancer at age 25 (It is possible). Sometimes patients delay visiting a doctor because they don't want to use an inhaler. Also, there are others who say they have never been ill before and that it couldn't happen to them. Few don't want to trouble their families with healthcare costs and be a burden on them, so they delay hospitalizations, and oftentimes they have young children to look after or important work to attend to. These, in my opinion, are reasons enough to sort out your health first because nothing can be a replacement for it.

The bottom line is that the earlier you consult a doctor, the sooner your problem can be identified, and it can be nipped much before it progresses to a more chronic version of the disease.

COUGH

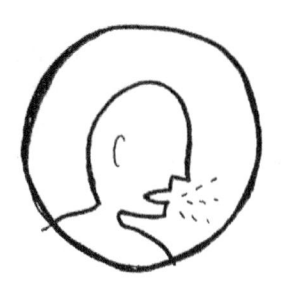

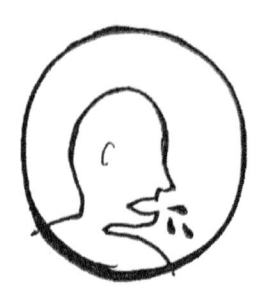

BLOOD IN SPUTUM

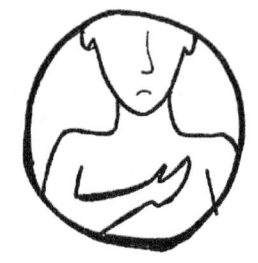

CHEST PAIN

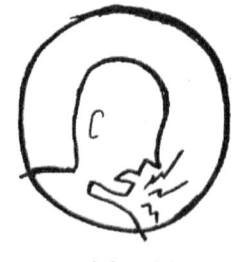

WHEEZING

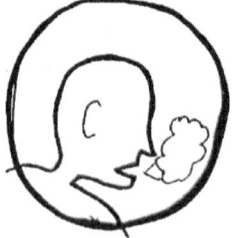

BREATHLESSNESS

You Are What You Breathe

There is a popular saying that 'You are what you eat'. I do agree. However, as a lung specialist, I must also tell you that you are what you breathe. If you inhale smoke, dust, fungal spores, and other toxic material, your lung health and, eventually, the quality of your life will be immensely affected. In this section, we will discuss the multiple scenarios and objects we come across in our daily lives which might be affecting us unknowingly and how we can prevent them.

Smoking 101

Everyone knows about the harmful effects of smoking. It is a leading cause of preventable death and disease worldwide. The side effects are numerous for both smokers and also for those exposed to second-hand smoke. It can cause cancer, affecting most body organs, and it is absolutely detrimental to the health of your lungs. Additionally, it shortens life expectancy by almost ten years as compared to non-smokers. If you are someone who smokes, you might want to pay attention.

Most patients that I see in my practice are well aware of all these effects. The problem, however, is with quitting. "I am unable to quit. I cannot quit, I have tried numerous times and failed." These are the most common things I have heard in my OPD.

Smoking exposes you to close to 7000 chemicals, of which about 70 have been identified to be carcinogens, which means that they can cause cancer. One of the most dangerous chemicals released is nicotine. It releases dopamine in our body which makes us feel good and thus makes us dependent. Nicotine shortens life expectancy. Once it fades away, the person will feel anxiety, nervousness, irritability, and difficulty in concentrating. Other chemicals like tar coat the lungs like soot. If you have been to a movie theatre in recent years, you would know this.

A smoker's lung, on autopsy, typically appears black and tar-like due to the build-up of tar and other chemicals from cigarette smoke. The lung tissue may also appear thickened and stiff, and the air spaces within the lung (alveoli) may be narrowed or blocked. Additionally, there may be areas of inflammation and scarring. Emphysema, a condition in which the air spaces in the lung are damaged and enlarged, is also commonly seen in a smoker's lung.

Smoking can cause lung cancer. According to the American Cancer Society, smoking is responsible for about 90% of lung cancer deaths in the United States. Additionally, smoking can increase the risk of other types of cancer, including throat, oesophagus, stomach, liver, colon, cervix, pancreas, bladder, and kidney cancer.

Other major effects of smoking are respiratory illnesses like COPD and the worsening of asthma. In the heart, it causes irregular heartbeat, raises blood pressure, and increases the risk of heart attack and stroke.

Smoking can also lead to problems with the immune system, making it harder for the body to fight off infections.

Additionally, smoking can cause damage to the eyes, leading to cataracts and age-related macular degeneration. It can lead to problems with fertility in both men and women and the fetus during pregnancy.

So let me begin by telling you first how soon the adverse effects start to wean away after quitting smoking. The good news is that when someone stops smoking, the body immediately begins to repair itself. Yes, that's right.

According to CDC (Centre for disease control), within 20 minutes of the last cigarette, the heart rate and blood pressure begin to normalize, and within eight hours, the carbon monoxide levels in the blood decrease to normal. After 24 hours, the heart attack risk decreases. In 48 hours, your nerve endings adjust to the absence of nicotine, and you begin to regain your ability to taste and smell. After two weeks to three months, blood circulation and exercise tolerance improve. In about a year's time, cough and breathlessness begin to improve, and the risk of heart attack drops sharply. In about 10-15 years, the added risk of lung cancer is reduced by half, and in about 15 years, the risk of coronary artery disease is minimised.

Quitting smoking can be difficult, but there are many resources available to help:

- Cold turkey: This method involves quitting smoking abruptly, without the use of any aids or medications.
- Nicotine replacement therapy: Nicotine replacement therapy (NRT) involves using products such as gum, patches, or lozenges to help manage withdrawal symptoms.
- Medications: Prescription medications, such as bupropion and varenicline, can help reduce cravings and withdrawal symptoms.

- Behavioural therapy: This can include counselling, support groups, or other forms of therapy to help address the psychological aspects of smoking addiction.
- Combination approach: This approach involves using a combination of the above methods, such as NRT and behavioural therapy, to increase the chances of success.

Air Pollution

Living in one of the most polluted cities in the world, I often wonder what effects it will have on my children, especially because, at that age, the lungs are more susceptible to damage. Air pollution is a major environmental issue that affects the health and well-being of people around the world. It is caused by a variety of sources, including industrial facilities, power plants, transportation, and agriculture.

One of the main sources of air pollution is the burning of fossil fuels, such as coal, oil, and natural gas. Burning them releases harmful substances, including particulate matter, sulfur dioxide, nitrogen oxides, and greenhouse gases like carbon dioxide. These pollutants can have serious health effects, such as respiratory illness, heart disease, and cancer. Cars, trucks, and buses emit a variety of pollutants, including particulate matter, nitrogen oxides, and carbon monoxide. These emissions have a significant impact on air quality, particularly in urban areas where traffic is heavy. Agriculture is also a major source of air pollution, particularly from the use of pesticides and fertilizers.

Acid rain can damage crops, forests, and bodies of water. Ozone depletion can harm plants and animals and contribute to global warming.

Air pollution is measured using the Air Quality Index or the AQI. It is divided into six categories, and a value of less than 50 suggests good quality air, while a value of more than 300 suggests hazardous air quality. Usually, a value less than 100 is thought to be satisfactory. For sensitive individuals, a value greater than 150 is detrimental. Sensitive groups include pregnant women, the elderly, children, and people with existing respiratory illnesses.

There are several measures individuals and governments can take to reduce air pollution. One of the most effective ways is to reduce the use of fossil fuels by increasing the use of renewable energy sources, such as solar and wind power and encouraging the development and use of electric and hybrid vehicles, and investment in public transportation systems. Factories can install pollution control equipment, and farmers can use alternative pest control methods.

Individuals can also take steps to reduce their own contributions to air pollution. For example, they can drive less, use public transportation, or bike or walk instead. They can also reduce their use of pesticides and fertilizers in their own gardens and support local farmers who employ sustainable practices.

Here are a few ways to protect your lungs from air pollution. Sensitive people should pay particular attention to these:

- Stay indoors on days when AQI is high.
- Wear a mask or respirator to filter out pollutants when you have to be outside.
- Avoid strenuous outdoor activities on days when AQI is high.
- Keep windows and doors closed to prevent outdoor pollutants from entering your home.

- Support efforts to reduce air pollution, such as promoting the use of clean energy sources and stricter emissions standards for vehicles and industries.
- Support and promote a healthy lifestyle, such as regular exercise, healthy diet, and stress management, to help keep your lungs healthy.
- Keep your home and workplace clean and well-ventilated to reduce indoor air pollution.

Stress

We live in a high-pressure society, and in one way or another, stress has become a part of our lifestyle in many ways. It is a well-known fact that stress causes cardiac problems, including hypertension and heart attacks.

Stress can also have a negative impact on the lungs and respiratory system. When a person is under stress, the body's "fight or flight" response is activated. This causes an increase in heart rate, blood pressure, and breathing rate, which can make it harder to breathe. Several studies have shown that chronic stress exerts a general immunosuppressive effect that suppresses or withholds the body's ability to initiate a prompt, efficient immune reaction. It is attributed to the abundance of corticosteroids produced during chronic stress, which produces an imbalance in corticosteroid levels and weakens immunocompetence. This can lead to an imbalance and inefficiency of the entire immune response. This is consistence with the finding that as we get elder, we are prone to suffer from infection, cancer, hypersensitivity and autoimmunity. Thus, Chronic stress can also lead to changes in the lungs and airways that make them more susceptible to infections and inflammation.

In addition, stress can also lead to unhealthy habits such as smoking, which can cause lung damage and increases the risk of lung cancer. Also, Stress can lead to poor sleep quality, which can make it harder for the lungs to repair and regenerate.

It's important to manage stress through healthy habits such as regular exercise, a healthy diet, and stress management techniques such as meditation, yoga, or therapy.

Birds

Birds can affect the lungs in a few different ways. Some people may experience allergic reactions to feathers, dust, or droppings from birds, which can lead to sneezing, coughing, and difficulty breathing. These reactions are known as avian allergies.

Birds are also carriers of certain diseases that can affect the lungs, such as avian influenza (bird flu) and psittacosis (parrot fever). These diseases can be transmitted to humans through contact with infected birds or their droppings.

It's important to take precautions to reduce the risk of exposure to birds and their by-products, such as wearing a mask and gloves when cleaning bird cages or handling birds and avoiding contact with sick or dead birds. If you have a history of respiratory issues or allergies, it's especially important to be cautious around birds and to seek medical attention if you experience any symptoms of lung irritation or infection.

Incense sticks

Incense sticks, or agarbattis, are commonly used in religious and spiritual ceremonies, as well as for home fragrance. A typical composition of stick incense consists of 21% (by weight) of herbal and wood powder, 35% of fragrance material, 11% of adhesive powder, and 33% of bamboo stick. Incense smoke contains particulate matter (PM), gas products and many organic compounds. On average, incense burning produces particulates greater than 45 mg/g burned as compared to 10 mg/g burned for cigarettes. Incense burning also produces volatile organic compounds, such as benzene, toluene, and xylenes, as well as aldehydes and polycyclic aromatic hydrocarbons (PAHs).

One of the main concerns is the release of particulate matter, which can be inhaled into the lungs and potentially cause respiratory problems. Studies have found that burning incense can increase the levels of particulate matter in the air, particularly fine particulate matter (PM2.5), which can penetrate deep into the lungs and cause inflammation.

It can also release other harmful chemicals such as formaldehyde, benzene, and polycyclic aromatic hydrocarbons (PAHs). These chemicals can be toxic when inhaled and have been linked to a range of health problems, like airway dysfunction. It has been indicated to cause allergic contact dermatitis.

However, some types of incense sticks may be less harmful than others. For example, natural incense made from plant materials such as sandalwood or sage may be less harmful than synthetic incense made from chemicals.

Be mindful of the type of incense sticks you use. Also, it is essential to always burn them in a well-ventilated area to minimise exposure.

Flowering Plants

Pollen is a fine powdery substance produced by plants, which is necessary for the fertilization of other plants. In some people, exposure to pollen can lead to a range of respiratory problems.

Pollen allergies, also known as hay fever, are a common problem during the spring and summer months when plants are in bloom. They can cause sneezing, runny nose, itchy eyes, and congestion. In severe cases, exposure to pollen can also lead to asthma attacks, which can make it difficult to breathe. Pollen can be easily inhaled into the lungs. Once the immune system recognizes the pollen as a foreign invader, it releases histamine and other chemicals to fight it off. This leads to inflammation and narrowing of the airways, making it difficult to breathe. People with pollen allergies are more susceptible to these problems, but even healthy individuals can be affected by high levels of pollen in the air.

To minimise the effects of pollen on the lungs, it's important to be aware of the pollen count and to avoid being outdoors during times of high pollen levels. Wearing a mask can also help to filter out pollen particles. If you have a pollen allergy, take your allergy medication as prescribed by your doctor, and keep your windows and doors closed during the peak pollen season.

House Dust Mite

House dust mites are tiny arthropods that are commonly found in indoor environments, particularly in areas with high humidity, such as bedrooms and carpets. These bugs are invisible to the naked eye. These mites feed on the dead skin cells that we shed, and their faeces and body parts can cause allergic reactions in some individuals. It can lead to a range of respiratory problems, particularly in people with allergies or asthma. The proteins found in the faeces of house dust mites can trigger an immune response, leading to symptoms such as sneezing, runny nose, itchy eyes, and congestion. In people with asthma, exposure to house dust mites can also cause asthma attacks, making it difficult to breathe. Additionally, it can cause symptoms in people who were previously asymptomatic.

To reduce exposure to house dust mites and their allergens, it's important to keep indoor humidity levels low (below 50%) and to use a dehumidifier if necessary. Vacuuming and dusting regularly, using mattress and pillow covers that are specifically designed to prevent mites, and washing bedding in hot water (greater than 130°F) weekly can help to reduce the population of mites.

Desert Coolers

Desert coolers or evaporative coolers are a type of air conditioning system that cools air by blowing it over water-moistened pads. While desert coolers can be an efficient and cost-effective way to cool indoor spaces, there are potential concerns about their effects on the lungs.

One of the main concerns with desert coolers is the release of Particulate Matter (PM) into the air. The water-moistened pads in desert coolers can harbour microorganisms such as bacteria and mold, which can be released into the air along with the cooled air. Inhaling these microorganisms can lead to respiratory problems, particularly in people with allergies or asthma. It also increases indoor humidity, which can promote the growth of mold and other allergens. High humidity levels can also make it easier for pollutants to become trapped indoors and can worsen symptoms of asthma and allergies.

Recent studies have shown that desert coolers are one of the leading causes of another respiratory disease called hypersensitivity pneumonitis.

Regular maintenance and cleaning of desert coolers can also help to reduce the release of pollutants into the air. To minimise the effects of desert coolers on the lungs, it's important to choose the models with better filtration systems to maintain and clean the units regularly and to monitor the indoor humidity levels.

Air Conditioners

Air conditioners, like any other mechanical systems, can have the potential to harm the lungs if not properly maintained or installed. Air conditioners can recirculate pollutants and allergens that are already present in the indoor air, such as dust, mold, and bacteria. These pollutants can aggravate respiratory symptoms in people with asthma or allergies. The cool and humid environment created by air conditioners can provide a breeding ground for mold, which can release spores into the air that can cause respiratory diseases. They release chemical compounds such as refrigerants and PM, which can have negative effects on the lungs if inhaled in large amounts.

Regularly maintain and clean air conditioning units to prevent mold growth, filter replacement, and check for leaks. Proper installation of the units also plays a crucial role in preventing the release of pollutants and chemical compounds into the air.

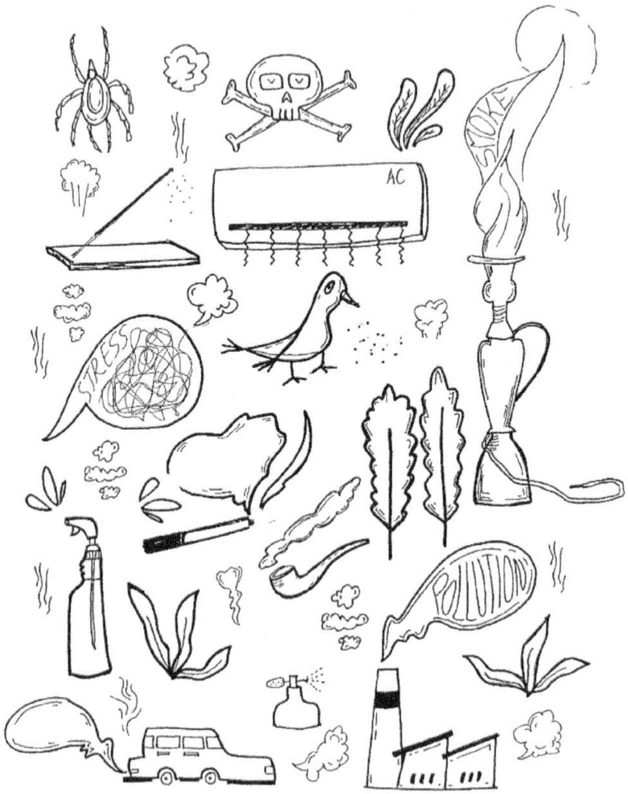
SMOKE
AC
STRESS
POLLUTION

Sleep and Lung Health: The Surprising Connection

Sleep is an essential component of overall health and well-being. Good sleep has numerous health benefits. Sleeping helps the brain to process memories and regulate emotions. It also promotes tissue repair and the release of proteins and hormones that help restore damaged tissues, including muscles. Additionally, sleep helps to boost the immune system function by producing cytokines which fight inflammation and reduce the risk of illnesses. However, in today's fast-paced world, many people prioritize work or other activities over sleep, resulting in sleep deprivation. The consequences of sleep deprivation can be severe and long-lasting, affecting both physical and mental health.

It can have both short-term and long-term consequences on our health. In the short term, lack of sleep can cause fatigue, mood disturbances, decreased attention and concentration, and impaired memory. In the long term, sleep deprivation can lead to an increased risk of chronic diseases such as obesity, diabetes, cardiovascular disease, and even early death. These effects are attributed to the disruption of the body's natural sleep-wake cycle, which affects hormone regulation, metabolism, and immune function.

Sleep disruption can be caused by a variety of factors, including lifestyle choices such as excessive caffeine or alcohol consumption, performing shift work, and exposure to light pollution. Stressful life circumstances like caregiving for a family member with a chronic illness or a young infant can also contribute to sleep problems. Medical conditions like obstructive sleep apnea and restless legs syndrome, as well as major medical conditions that require nighttime monitoring, have also been associated with sleep disruption. Sleep deprivation is a complex issue that involves a combination of biological, psychological, genetic, and social factors.

Maintaining good sleep hygiene is essential for a healthy and restful sleep. Sleep hygiene refers to the practices and habits that can promote healthy sleep. Here are some tips for maintaining good sleep hygiene:

- Stick to a consistent sleep schedule.
- Create a relaxing bedtime routine to signal to your body that it's time to sleep.
- Use comfortable bedding and pillows, and invest in a supportive mattress
- Make sure your sleep environment is dark, cool, and quiet.
- Avoid stimulating activities before bed, such as watching TV or using electronic devices.
- Limit caffeine and alcohol intake, especially before bedtime.
- Avoid large meals and excessive fluid intake before bed.
- Exercise regularly, but avoid intense workouts close to bedtime.

- Manage stress through relaxation techniques like meditation or deep breathing exercises.
- If you can't fall asleep within 20-30 minutes, get up and do a relaxing activity until you feel sleepy.
- Consider seeking medical help if you have persistent sleep problems.

Sleep apnea is underdiagnosed in our part of the world. Mainly the reason being the non-recognition of its symptoms as being a problem. Sleep apnea is a sleep disorder in which breathing stops and starts repeatedly while you sleep. To prevent this from harming the body and to maintain oxygen levels in your body, the brain wakes you up to breathe, and this results in repeated waking up during the night. Sometimes these awakenings are so short that you may not even remember them. What results is what we call non-restorative sleep, which means you wake up feeling tired and unrested. Sleep apnea can be mild, moderate, or severe and pose serious health risks if not attended to in a timely manner.

Fatigue and tiredness are common symptoms of sleep apnea, along with snoring and excessive daytime sleepiness, but they are often missed by unsuspecting people.

October 2015

A 50-year-old man, Rajeev, had been struggling with loud snoring and tiredness for years. He came to my OPD with his wife, Smita, who was bothered by his snoring disorder, so much so that she had decided to sleep in a different room for the past few months. Rajeev thought his wife was making a big deal out of this. He had always assumed that it was just a normal part of aging, and he never thought to seek medical attention. However, things changed when one day, he was driving back from work and fell asleep at the wheels of his car. It must have been for a few seconds, but when he woke up, he was in the middle of a cross-section surrounded by cars and horns were blaring. He was stunned. This had never happened before.

I told him his symptoms were a classic case of sleep apnea. Rajeev needed a sleep study and a few more tests before we began treatment.

During a sleep study, several sensors are attached to the person's body to measure different aspects of their sleep, such as brain activity, eye movement, heart rate, breathing patterns, and muscle movement. The person then sleeps in the lab or at home, with the sensors recording data throughout the night. The next day, a sleep specialist reviews the data and assesses the person's sleep patterns to determine if they have a sleep disorder and develops a treatment plan if needed.

Rajeev was shocked to learn that his snoring was a sign of a serious health problem, and he was even more surprised to learn that his sleep apnea was putting him at risk for lung problems. He was determined to take control of his health. He underwent a sleep study and began using his Continuous Positive Airway Pressure (CPAP) machine every night.

On his visit after about one and a half months, I reviewed his reports. His sleep apnea improved, and he started to feel more rested and alert during the day. He also stopped smoking and lost weight, which further helped to improve his lung health. Smita was glad his condition had improved. She was sleeping as peacefully as him now in the same room.

The most common symptoms of sleep apnea are:

- Snoring
- Excessive daytime sleepiness
- Fatigue
- Morning headaches

- Observed breathing disturbance at night by the partner, Choking episodes
- Mood changes

Oftentimes, these symptoms are dismissed as tiredness or stress.

Sleep apnea could be either Obstructive, central, or mixed. Obstructive Sleep Apnea (OSA) is the more common variant, where the throat muscles collapse and block the flow of air from the nose into the lungs. Central Sleep Apnea (CSA) occurs when the brain fails to send accurate signals to the muscles to control breathing. Mixed apnea is a combination of the two.

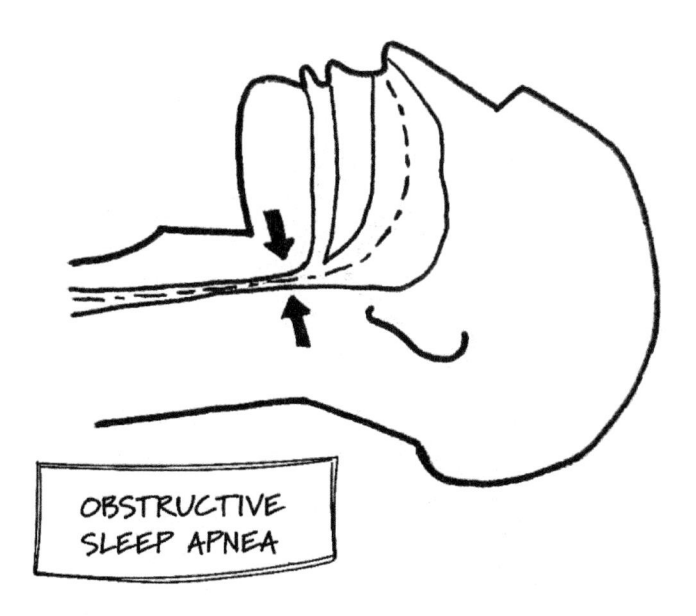

OBSTRUCTIVE SLEEP APNEA

Patients with OSA have recurrent airway obstruction. This will cause an increase in heart rate and a rise in blood pressure during these events due to a strain on the heart through the night. The awakenings end the airway occlusion and are accompanied by a sympathetic nervous system response. Multiple studies have found OSAS patients to be at an increased risk for cardiac complications and hypertension.

Other consequences are metabolic diseases such as diabetes, stroke, depression, and increased surgical complications. It also results in increased errors in the workplace, traffic accidents, and untimely deaths.

Saavi was a 35-year-old woman who had been struggling with asthma for years. She had always assumed that her asthma was just a chronic condition that she would have to live with for the rest of her life. She did not have the typical symptoms of OSA, and neither did she fit the profile of a person with OSA, though she was diagnosed with sleep apnea, which was causing her asthma symptoms to worsen.

She was prescribed a CPAP machine and instructed to use it every night. She was amazed at the difference it made in her asthma symptoms. She no longer had to rely on her rescue inhaler as often and was able to enjoy a better quality of life.

The learning point here is that when a patient has an existing respiratory illness that is not getting controlled by medications, it is a good idea to explore other potential causes of nonresponse to treatment or worsening condition.

The main treatment for OSA is a CPAP device. It delivers air at a fixed pressure to keep the airways open while you sleep and prevents airway collapse. A hose connects the machine (which generates the pressure) on one end and the mask on the other end. The mask is then attached to your mouth and nose or nose.

Mild OSA is treated with lifestyle changes, including weight loss and exercise. Also, it is essential to limit alcohol intake and avoid sedatives and anti-anxiety medicines before bedtime. Another popular method is to sleep on your side rather than your back to prevent the muscles of the throat and tongue from falling back and narrowing/blocking your air passage.

Moderate to severe OSA treatment requires the use of CPAP machines. Often times a Bilevel machine might be required.

In some cases, you may also be able to use a special mouthguard that helps keep your airways open while you sleep. An oral appliance is a type of mouthguard that you wear while you sleep. It's designed to help reposition your tongue and jaw, which can help keep your airway open and prevent interruptions in breathing. This is a less invasive option for people with sleep apnea compared to using a CPAP machine or having surgery.

In some severe cases, however, surgery may be recommended. There are a couple of different surgical options that can help treat sleep apnea. One is called uvulopalato-pharyngoplasty (UPPP), which involves removing the excess tissue from the mouth and throat that can block the airway. Another option is called genioglossus advancement (GA), which involves moving the tongue forward to keep the airway open.

It's important to know that not everyone with sleep apnea will need surgery, and most people will be able to manage their condition with a combination of lifestyle changes and CPAP therapy or an oral appliance. A sleep specialist will be able to help determine the best course of treatment for you based on the severity of your sleep apnea and your individual needs.

Often, I get asked questions in day-to-day conversations with patients and their caregivers or even my own family and friends about some common myths and facts about lung diseases. I have addressed these in the next section.

Clearing the Air: Dispelling Myths Around Lung Diseases

October 2018

It was a winter Monday morning. I was sitting in my OPD when a mother walked in with her 14-year-old boy. The boy was coughing, and his mother was clearly distraught. She told me he had been coughing for the past one week. He avoided playing as much as he used to, slept poorly at night, and she said she often heard a sound while he breathed, especially at night. What she described was wheezing. A detailed history revealed she had already shown two other doctors for his symptoms that very week. He had a past history of similar episodes during winters. I examined him, and it was clear he was wheezing. I looked at all his reports and the chest X-ray which was done for him.

"He has Asthma," I said.

"Yes, I was told so, but I don't want him to take inhalers. Can you give him some medicine?" Said the mother.

"Well, Inhalers are the recommended treatment. Why don't you want him to take it?" I questioned.

"Doctor, he is still young. I don't want him to be dependent on inhalers. These contain steroids, I have read. Once it is started, he will continue to for all his life," she exclaimed.

Well, this was not the first time I was hearing this, so I wasn't surprised when she said it.

"Inhalers are not addictive. They contain medication that helps to open up the airways and make it easier to breathe. When used as prescribed, inhalers are a safe and effective treatment for asthma. Inhaled steroids are the recommended treatment for asthma. There are no oral medicines which can treat his symptoms effectively. I strongly recommend you start his treatment as soon as possible to prevent his asthma to convert from a treatable version to a more advanced stage," I reassured her.

This is just another day in the OPD. There are so many myths surrounding respiratory diseases, and these lead to delays in treatments and sometimes even no treatment at all.

In this chapter, we'll be diving deep into the world of lung conditions, separating fact from fiction. From old wives' tales about food and respiratory diseases to misconceptions about inhalers and ventilators, I'll be busting the myths and leaving behind the confusion and misinformation.

Some of the common myths are discussed here.

Cold weather causes respiratory infections.

It is a misconception that cold weather causes respiratory infections. Cold weather doesn't cause respiratory infections, but it can make it more likely for people to catch them. People tend to spend more time indoors in cold weather and in close proximity to each other, which makes it easier for germs to spread.

You can catch a cold from being cold.

It is untrue that you can catch a cold from being cold. Cold is caused by viruses, and these viruses are spread through the air when an infected person coughs or sneezes or by touching a surface that has the virus on it and then touching your face.

Antibiotics can cure common cold.
Antibiotics only work against bacterial infections, not viral infections like the common cold. Taking antibiotics when you have a cold can actually do more harm than good because it can lead to antibiotic resistance, where antibiotics become less effective over time.

You only need to wear a mask if you're sick.
Wearing a mask can help protect you and others from getting sick, whether you're sick or not. When you wear a mask, you're less likely to spread the virus if you're infected, and you're also less likely to inhale the virus if someone else is infected.

If you have no symptoms, your lungs are healthy
Some lung diseases, such as Chronic Obstructive Pulmonary Disease (COPD) and lung cancer, may not show symptoms in the early stages. It is important to get regular check-ups and screenings, especially if you have risk factors such as a history of smoking.

Only older people or people with underlying health conditions are at risk of respiratory infections
Anyone can catch a respiratory infection, regardless of their age or health status. While older adults and people with underlying health conditions may be at a higher risk of complications from a respiratory infection, it's important for everyone to take precautions to protect themselves and others.

You can't spread a respiratory infection once you have no symptoms
It's possible to spread a respiratory infection before you have symptoms and even after your symptoms have gone away. People who are infected with a virus can be contagious for several days before they feel sick, and in some cases, they can continue to be contagious for a week or more after they recover.

You only need to worry about respiratory infections during cold and flu season

Respiratory infections can happen at any time of the year. Though the common cold and the flu(Influenza virus) are more common during the fall and winter months, other types of respiratory infections (caused by adenovirus, human bocavirus, human metapneumovirus (hMPV), and rhinovirus) can occur throughout the year.

Steam inhalation with hot water can help cure a cold

Steam inhalation can help relieve nasal congestion, but it won't cure a cold. A cold is caused by a virus, and antibiotics are not effective against viruses. Steam inhalation can also be harmful if the water is too hot, as it can burn the nasal passages.

Eating spicy food can cause asthma

Eating spicy food does not cause asthma. However, it's possible that spicy food can trigger asthma symptoms in some people. If you have asthma and find that spicy food triggers your symptoms, you may want to limit your intake or avoid spicy foods altogether.

Vitamin C can prevent cold

Vitamin C can't prevent cold, but it may help to shorten the duration of a cold if taken at the onset of symptoms. While vitamin C can help boost the immune system, it's not a cure for common cold.

Consuming a lot of antioxidants can prevent respiratory infections

Consuming a diet rich in antioxidants may help to support overall health and boost the immune system, but it is not proven to prevent respiratory infections. Eating a balanced diet with a variety of fruits, vegetables, and lean proteins is always recommended to support a healthy immune system.

Eating dairy products can increase mucus production and make respiratory infections worse

Eating dairy products doesn't increase mucus production. In fact, studies have shown that there is no link between dairy consumption and increased mucus production.

Eating garlic can prevent respiratory infections.

Garlic has antimicrobial properties, but it is not proven to prevent respiratory infections. While it's healthy food and can be included in a balanced diet, it is not a magic bullet for preventing respiratory infections.

Only smokers get lung cancer

While smoking is the leading risk factor for lung cancer, people who have never smoked can also develop the disease. Exposure to radon, air pollution, and certain chemicals can also increase the risk of lung cancer.

There is no cure for lung disease

While there is no cure for some lung diseases, such as emphysema, there are treatments that can help manage the symptoms and improve the quality of life.

You can't regain lung function

While it is true that lung damage is irreversible, quitting smoking and other lifestyle changes can help slow the progression of lung disease and improve lung function.

If you have lung disease, you should avoid exercise

Exercise can help people with lung disease by improving their lung function and overall health. Therefore, it is essential to engage in regular moderate exercise even if you have a lung disease after consultation with your doctor.

Inhalers are only for people with severe asthma
Inhalers are a common treatment for asthma, and they can be used for people with mild, moderate, or severe asthma. Inhalers can help to open up the airways and make it easier to breathe.

Inhalers have a lot of side effects
Inhalers can have some side effects, but they are generally mild. The most common side effects of inhalers are a dry or sore throat, a hoarse voice, and a bad taste in the mouth.

You only need to use an inhaler when you're having an asthma attack
It's important to use an inhaler as directed by your healthcare provider, even when you're not having an asthma attack. Preventer inhalers are typically used on a regular basis to help prevent asthma symptoms from occurring in the first place.

Chemotherapy is the only treatment option for lung cancer
Chemotherapy is one treatment option for lung cancer, but it's not the only option. Other treatment options for lung cancer include radiation therapy, surgery, targeted therapy, and immunotherapy. The best treatment plan for an individual with lung cancer will depend on the stage of the cancer and the overall health of the patient.

Ventilators are only used for people who are near death
Ventilators are used to help people who have difficulty breathing, regardless of their overall health status. People who are critically ill or have severe respiratory infections may need a

ventilator to help them breathe, but the machine can also be used to assist people who have chronic lung conditions such as COPD or asthma or to help people who need to be sedated for surgery.

Once you're on a ventilator, you'll never be able to breathe on your own again

Many people who are on a ventilator are able to wean off the machine and breathe on their own again. The length of time a person needs to be on a ventilator depends on the individual's condition and the underlying cause of their respiratory distress.

In conclusion, there are many myths and misconceptions about day-to-day practices and respiratory diseases such as COPD, asthma, and lung cancer. It's important to separate fact from fiction when it comes to these illnesses in order to make informed decisions about our health.

It's important to remember that while some foods and supplements may have a positive effect on our overall health and immune system, they cannot prevent or cure respiratory diseases. Also, while ventilators can be life-saving for people with difficulty breathing, they are not always necessary, or they are dangerous.

It's always a good idea to consult with a healthcare professional to get the facts and to develop a personalized plan that is tailored to your needs and health conditions. Therefore, always be vigilant, try to get accurate information from credible sources, and don't hesitate to ask questions. Remember that knowledge is power, and being informed can help you make better decisions about your health and well-being, as well as that of your loved ones.

(PART THREE)

BEYOND THE PANDEMIC

The COVID-19 Pandemic: Reflections and Lessons

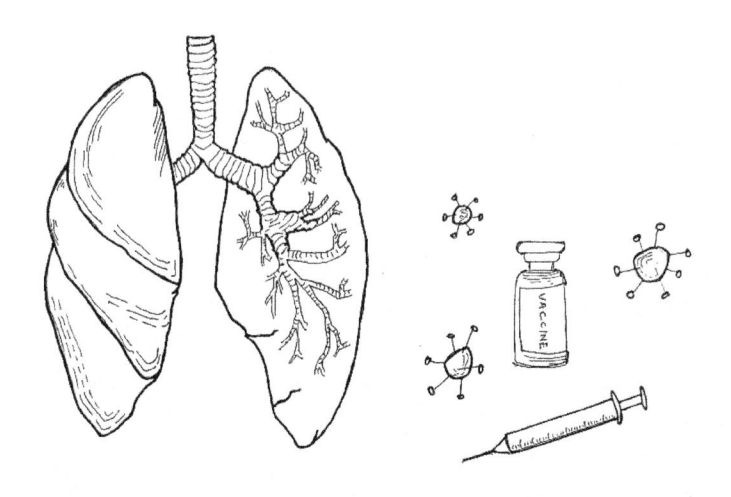

March 2020

Early morning before work would begin, I loved to sit at the dining table with my coffee and my newspaper. There was news of a new virus spreading across the world. It was thought to have started in China. It was alarming to see the rate at which the virus was spreading. I thought a respiratory virus that is so virulent was really going to be difficult to control.

Reported cases of respiratory virus in India were very few prior to the outbreak of the pandemic. Therefore, there were no clear-cut guidelines or treatment strategies yet. It was scary. If the developed world was struggling to keep up with this virus, how would we over-power it?

I remember the first patient I treated who had Covid-19. A 55-year-old woman was brought into the hospital with severe symptoms. She was struggling to breathe, and her oxygen levels were dangerously low. The team immediately sprang into action, to stabilize her condition and begin treatment.

She was frightened because she knew about how this virus was causing havoc around the world. She was isolated and unable to see her family members. Even the staff treating her was always dressed in PPE (Personal Protective Equipment). The feeling of being isolated and the scare of death is enough to demoralize anyone.

Despite the challenges presented by the virus, we were determined to save her life. Gradually, oxygenation began to improve, and she started to feel better. Ultimately, ten days later, she was discharged with some residual lung fibrosis.

However, I knew that the battle against COVID-19 was far from over. I continued to see more and more patients with the virus and knew that we would have to work tirelessly on the front lines to save as many lives as possible.

This pandemic has certainly been a wild ride, hasn't it? We've all had to adjust to a new way of living, and it hasn't been easy. But even in the midst of all this craziness, there are valuable lessons we can take away from this experience. From how we handle healthcare to how we handle remote work, the pandemic has given us a unique opportunity to re-evaluate and improve our healthcare systems.

In this chapter, we'll delve into some of the lessons from the pandemic and how we can use them to shape a brighter future. It may have been a tough journey, but let's make sure we come out of it stronger and more equipped to handle whatever comes our way in the future. These lessons can be extrapolated and applied to our lives in general.

Lesson 1: Prepare for the unexpected

Being prepared for the unexpected allows you to respond quickly and effectively to unforeseen events, minimizing the potential negative impact and maximizing the chances of a positive outcome. It also helps to reduce stress and anxiety, as you are better equipped to handle unexpected situations. Additionally, being prepared can help you to identify and take advantage of opportunities that arise unexpectedly. Having emergency plans in place is important because it helps to ensure that people and organizations can respond quickly and effectively to unexpected and potentially dangerous situations. It also minimizes confusion and chaos. So always prepare mentally, physically, and financially.

Lesson 2: Health is wealth

This is an age-old saying. If you take care of your body, your body takes care of you in the long run. Watch what you eat, exercise regularly, and maintain a good sleep routine. Avoid alcohol, tobacco, and other drugs. These are just the basics to minimize the need to visit a physician. Get regular health check-ups and screening tests as recommended for you by your doctor. Old age will not seem so isolating and debilitating if health is by your side. And not just physical health. This pandemic has taught us the importance of mental health as well. Isolation and loneliness are worrisome, and it might not just be an old age thing. It affects everyone. Manage stress levels by meditating and being mindful. Ask for help.

The pandemic has also shown the need to have well-funded and well-staffed healthcare facilities to handle a surge in patients and ensure everyone gets the care they need so that we are ready for whatever comes our way.

Lesson 3: Change is inevitable

Lots of people were left unemployed, salaries were halved, and millions fell sick. The scale of this virus was not anticipated. Most companies shifted to a work from home model, and a lot of companies shut down.

No matter how much you plan, things can change. Be open to changes and more willing to adapt to new situations quickly and keep your options open. When you face unexpected challenges, and life takes a pivot, explore new grounds and new areas. You never know what's in store. It is ultimately up to us to decide how we react to change. With an open mind and a positive attitude, we can turn change into an opportunity for growth and progress.

Lesson 4: Declutter your life

Life is really simple. We all have basic needs, and everything above that is a want. It is a luxury. There is no end to our wants. Minimize the clutter in your life to understand what is really important. It could be cluttered due to things or the clutter of thoughts in your mind. Once you minimize these, you realize things are not as complicated as we make them out to be. Live in the present rather than dwelling in the past or romanticizing the future. Live in the moment and enjoy the little things in life.

Lesson 5: No one is safe until everyone is safe

The pandemic has shown us this. To effectively fight a global crisis, we must come together and cooperate on a global scale. International cooperation is essential in order to ensure that resources and information are shared and that the most vulnerable are protected.

While the pandemic has been a difficult time, we can learn from it and come out stronger. By applying the lessons we've learned, we can create a more resilient society.

The Aftermath: Post Covid-19 Syndrome

February 2021

"Doctor, I am really tired of coming to the hospital again and again. You said I have recovered from covid. But I don't feel like I am back to being myself. I used to be so active. Now I can barely walk one flight of stairs, and I get breathless," said Radhika.

Radhika is a 35year old woman. I first saw her when she came to the hospital's emergency room with oxygen levels of 80%. She was gasping for breath, unable to even utter a single word. We had to admit her to the ICU. Her oxygen levels fluctuated as low as 65% with movement. She was on high-flow oxygen for nearly a month. She stayed in the ICU for nearly two weeks. Once her oxygen requirement was reduced to 2-3 lit of oxygen, we transferred her to the room. Frankly speaking, the CT scan of her lungs was so bad that it did not seem at one point that we would be able to save her life. Seeing her today in my OPD today felt like such an achievement to me.

But, of course, it did not seem like that to her. She was hoping for a complete recovery when she was discharged. She wanted to go back to her routine—her normal life, which meant normal activities, work, running errands, and socializing. But everything was leaving her tired. I did tell her it would take time before she would be her normal self, and she might even have to live with some lung fibrosis.

Three months after she was discharged, she returned with complaints of breathing difficulty and suffocation. I was not surprised as she was not the first patient to have experienced these symptoms. Radhika was clearly distraught, likely anyone who would be in her position. I did not have much to offer her except some breathing exercises and asking her to enrol in a pulmonary rehabilitation program. She also agreed to take medication, normally for some pulmonary fibrosis patients, which might improve her lung capacity, but the benefit of which is not clearly proven in covid induced pulmonary fibrosis.

The good news is that most people who get COVID-19 will experience mild to moderate symptoms and will recover without any long-term effects. However, some people who have had severe COVID-19 may experience ongoing problems even after they've recovered.

It has been found that such adverse outcomes do not affect only our lungs. Different organs can have long-term effects on different patients. In some, it affects the immune system, causing syndromes like Guillain–Barré syndrome, rheumatoid arthritis, and paediatric inflammatory multisystem syndromes such as Kawasaki disease. It might also cause slowing of the flow of blood in vessels and blood clots in others, and the heart might be involved while causing thickening of heart muscles – myocardial hypertrophy, blockage of heart's blood supply- coronary artery atherosclerosis, heart muscle thickening – focal myocardial fibrosis, or acute stoppage of blood to the heart- acute myocardial infarction. In few people, there can be long-term effects such as diarrhoea, nausea/vomiting, abdominal pain, loss of appetite, acid reflux, gastrointestinal bleeding, constipation, skin diseases, loss of taste/smell/hearing, headaches, spasms, convulsions, confusion, visual impairment, nerve pain, dizziness, impaired consciousness, stroke, brain haemorrhage and in many it can lead to stress, depression, and anxiety.

However, the most common long-term effect has been seen in the lungs and the respiratory system. This includes respiratory failure, pulmonary embolism or clots, and pulmonary fibrosis.

One of the main ways that COVID-19 affects the lungs is by causing inflammation. Any lung injury is followed by acute inflammation as well as an attempt at repair. This process can result in the restoration of normal lung architecture, or it may lead to lung fibrosis with architectural distortion and irreversible lung dysfunction. This can lead to the formation of scar tissue, which can make it harder for the lungs to function properly. Additionally, it can result in ongoing breathing problems, such as shortness of breath and fatigue. In some cases, this can even lead to interstitial lung disease or pulmonary fibrosis. The symptoms are prolonged dry cough, breathlessness, fatigue, or low oxygen levels.

Also, COVID-19 affects the lungs by causing blood clots. In severe cases, these clots can travel to the lungs and cause a condition called pulmonary embolism. This can be very serious and can lead to a range of symptoms, including shortness of breath, chest pain, and rapid or irregular heartbeat.

It's important to remember that not everyone who gets COVID-19 will experience lung problems. However, people who smoke, excessively drink alcohol, have a pre-existing lung condition, are older, have had a severe lung infection resulting from COVID, were admitted to the ICU (intensive care unit), or were mechanically ventilated are at a higher risk of developing lung problems after having COVID-19.

Until now, there is no specific therapy to handle post-inflammatory pulmonary fibrosis due to COVID-19 infection. Some anti-fibrotic medications have been used in trials and are under research; however, sufficient data is still not available about their efficacy.

So how should you help your lungs recover from COVID-19?

Here are some tips:

Get vaccinated: This is one of the most important things you can do to protect yourself from COVID-19. The vaccines have been shown to be highly effective in preventing severe illness and hospitalization.

Practice good hygiene: Wash your hands frequently, wear a mask, and avoid close contact with people who are sick.

Avoid smoking: If you smoke, now is the time to quit. Smoking can make your lungs more vulnerable to the effects of COVID-19.

Get a pulse oximeter and monitor your oxygen levels. Maintain a diary and enter values so your doctor can examine them.

Pulmonary rehabilitation is a multidisciplinary intervention based on personalised evaluation and treatment, which includes exercise training, education, and behavioural modification to improve the physical and psychological condition of people with respiratory disease.

The breathing pattern may be altered, with reduced diaphragmatic movement and greater use of neck and shoulder accessory muscles after any prolonged illness. This results in shallow breathing, fatigue and shortness of breath, and higher energy expenditure.

The "breathing control" technique is aimed at normalising breathing patterns and increasing the efficiency of the respiratory muscles (including the diaphragm). This will result in less energy expenditure, fatigue, and improvement in breathlessness.

The patient should sit in a supported position and breathe in and out slowly, breathing in through the nose and out through the mouth while relaxing the chest and shoulders and allowing the tummy to rise. They should aim for an inspiration to expiration ratio of 1:2. This technique can be used frequently throughout the day in 5-10 minute bursts.

COVID-19 has had a significant impact on lung health and other critical systems of our body. It is important to identify any symptoms early on and consult your doctor because sometimes we don't think a nagging symptom like a headache or a cough or non-specific pain in the abdomen is worth getting checked, but it might be a post-COVID sequela. It might be easily treatable too wit some home remedies, medication, or exercises.

As I conclude this book, I want to take a moment to reflect on why I wrote this book for you. For me, the decision to write this book was driven by a desire to educate and inform about the importance of respiratory health and the factors that can impact lung function. I also wanted to raise awareness about lung diseases and inspire people to take action to protect their respiratory health and advocate for cleaner air and healthier environments.

Whether you are a healthcare professional, a patient, a caregiver, or simply someone who cares about their respiratory health, I hope that this book has provided you with valuable insights and practical tips for maintaining healthy lungs.

Throughout this book, we have explored the intricate workings of the respiratory system, from the anatomy of the lungs to the process of breathing and gas exchange. We have delved into the various factors that can impact lung health, including environmental pollutants, lifestyle choices, and genetic predispositions, and the potential consequences of ignoring these factors.

We have seen that respiratory diseases can have a significant impact on quality of life and overall health, ranging from mild symptoms to life-threatening conditions. However, we have also seen that many respiratory diseases are preventable or treatable with the right interventions, emphasizing the importance of early detection and treatment.

I have emphasized the importance of taking proactive steps to maintain healthy lungs and prevent respiratory diseases. From quitting smoking and reducing exposure to pollutants to exercising regularly and maintaining a healthy diet, there are many practical and effective strategies that can help promote respiratory health.

Overall, my goal in writing this book is to empower you with the knowledge and tools needed to take control of your respiratory health and improve your overall well-being. I hope that this book has served as a constrictive resource for you and that you will continue to prioritize your lung health and advocate for a healthier world.

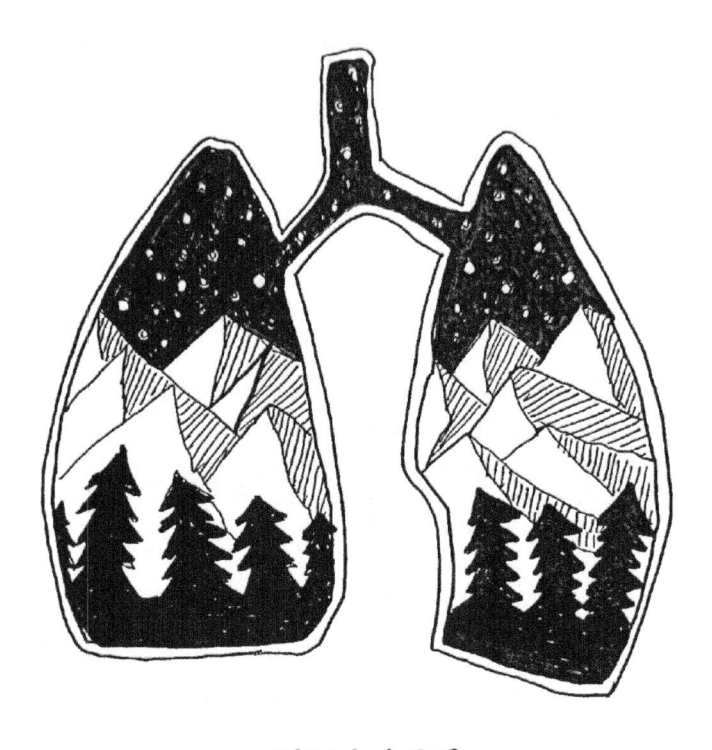

YOU ARE
what you breathe

About the Author

Pallavi Periwal is a pulmonologist. She completed her DNB in Respiratory Medicine from India and was awarded the prestigious Dr M. Santhosham Gold Medal award. She has studied medicine and worked as a doctor in India, Nepal, the USA, and the United Kingdom, bringing her expertise and compassion to people from all walks of life. She now resides in the UK with her amazing husband and her lovely son. She loves spending time with her family, exploring the local countryside, and delving into a good book while sipping coffee from a big mug. This is her first book.

Notes

Here are some scientific papers, books, articles, and online resources that can help you delve deeper into the ideas and concepts discussed in the book. This list is not exhaustive, will serve as a helpful starting point to adopt a new outlook and put into practice the principles of making every breath count.

1. Schittny JC. Development of the lung. Cell Tissue Res. 2017;367(3):427-444. doi:10.1007/s00441-016-2545-0
2. Bocci V. (2011). The potential toxicity of ozone: side effects and contraindications of ozone therapy, in Ozone: A New Medical Drug (Dordrecht: Springer)75–84
3. Misra A, Chowbey P, Makkar BM, Vikram NK, Wasir JS, Chadha D, Joshi SR, Sadikot S, Gupta R, Gulati S, Munjal YP; Concensus Group. Consensus statement for diagnosis of obesity, abdominal obesity, and the metabolic syndrome for Asian Indians and recommendations for physical activity, medical and surgical management. J Assoc Physicians India. 2009 Feb;57:163-70. PMID: 19582986.

4. Brock JM, Billeter A, Müller-Stich BP, Herth F. Obesity and the Lung: What We Know Today. Respiration. 2020;99(10):856-866.
5. https://www.lung.org/lung-health-diseases
6. Your lungs and exercise. Breathe (Sheff). 2016 Mar;12(1):97-100. doi: 10.1183/20734735.ELF121. PMID: 27066145; PMCID: PMC4818249.
7. https://www.nhs.uk/conditions/vaccinations/pneumococcal-vaccination/
8. https://www.nhs.uk/conditions/vaccinations/flu-influenza-vaccine/
9. Irwin RS, French CL, Chang AB, Altman KW; CHEST Expert Cough Panel*. Classification of Cough as a Symptom in Adults and Management Algorithms: CHEST Guideline and Expert Panel Report. Chest. 2018 Jan;153(1):196-209.
10. Oduwole O, Udoh EE, Oyo-Ita A, Meremikwu MM. Honey for acute cough in children. Cochrane Database Syst Rev. 2018 Apr 10;4(4):CD007094.
11. https://www.nhsinform.scot/illnesses-and-conditions/lungs-and-airways/cough
12. Donald A. Mahler; Denis E. O'Donnell (2014). Dyspnea: Mechanisms, Measurement, and Management, Third Edition. CRC Press. p. 3. ISBN 978-1-4822-0869-6
13. https://www.cancer.org/cancer/risk-prevention/tobacco/health-risks-of-tobacco/health-risks-of-smoking-tobacco.html
14. https://www.cancer.gov/about-cancer/causes-prevention/risk/tobacco/cessation-fact-sheet
15. Manisalidis I, Stavropoulou E, Stavropoulos A, Bezirtzoglou E. Environmental and Health Impacts of Air Pollution: A Review. Front Public Health. 2020 Feb

20;8:14. doi: 10.3389/fpubh.2020.00014. PMID: 32154200; PMCID: PMC7044178.
16. **https://www.asthmaandlung.org**
17. Salleh MR. Life event, stress and illness. Malays J Med Sci. 2008 Oct;15(4):9-18. PMID: 22589633; PMCID: PMC3341916.
18. Lin TC, Krishnaswamy G, Chi DS. Incense smoke: clinical, structural and molecular effects on airway disease. Clin Mol Allergy. 2008 Apr 25;6:3. doi: 10.1186/1476-7961-6-3. PMID: 18439280; PMCID: PMC2377255.
19. **https://acaai.org/allergies/allergic-conditions/dust-allergies/**
20. Medic G, Wille M, Hemels ME. Short- and long-term health consequences of sleep disruption. Nat Sci Sleep. 2017 May 19;9:151-161. doi: 10.2147/NSS.S134864. PMID: 28579842; PMCID: PMC5449130.
21. **https://healthysleep.med.harvard.edu/need-sleep/whats-in-it-for-you/health**
22. https://health.clevelandclinic.org/sleep-and-health/
23. Slowik JM, Sankari A, Collen JF. Obstructive Sleep Apnea. 2022 Dec 11. In: StatPearls [Internet]. Treasure Island (FL): StatPearls Publishing; 2023 Jan–. PMID: 29083619.
24. Lopez-Leon S, Wegman-Ostrosky T, Perelman C, Sepulveda R, Rebolledo PA, Cuapio A, Villapol S. More than 50 Long-term effects of COVID-19: a systematic review and meta-analysis. medRxiv [Preprint]. 2021 Jan 30:2021.01.27.21250617. doi: 10.1101/2021.01.27.21250617. Update in: Sci Rep. 2021 Aug 9;11(1):16144. PMID: 33532785; PMCID: PMC7852236.

25. Joshee S, Vatti N, Chang C. Long-Term Effects of COVID-19. Mayo Clin Proc. 2022 Mar;97(3):579-599. doi: 10.1016/j.mayocp.2021.12.017. Epub 2022 Jan 12. PMID: 35246288; PMCID: PMC8752286.

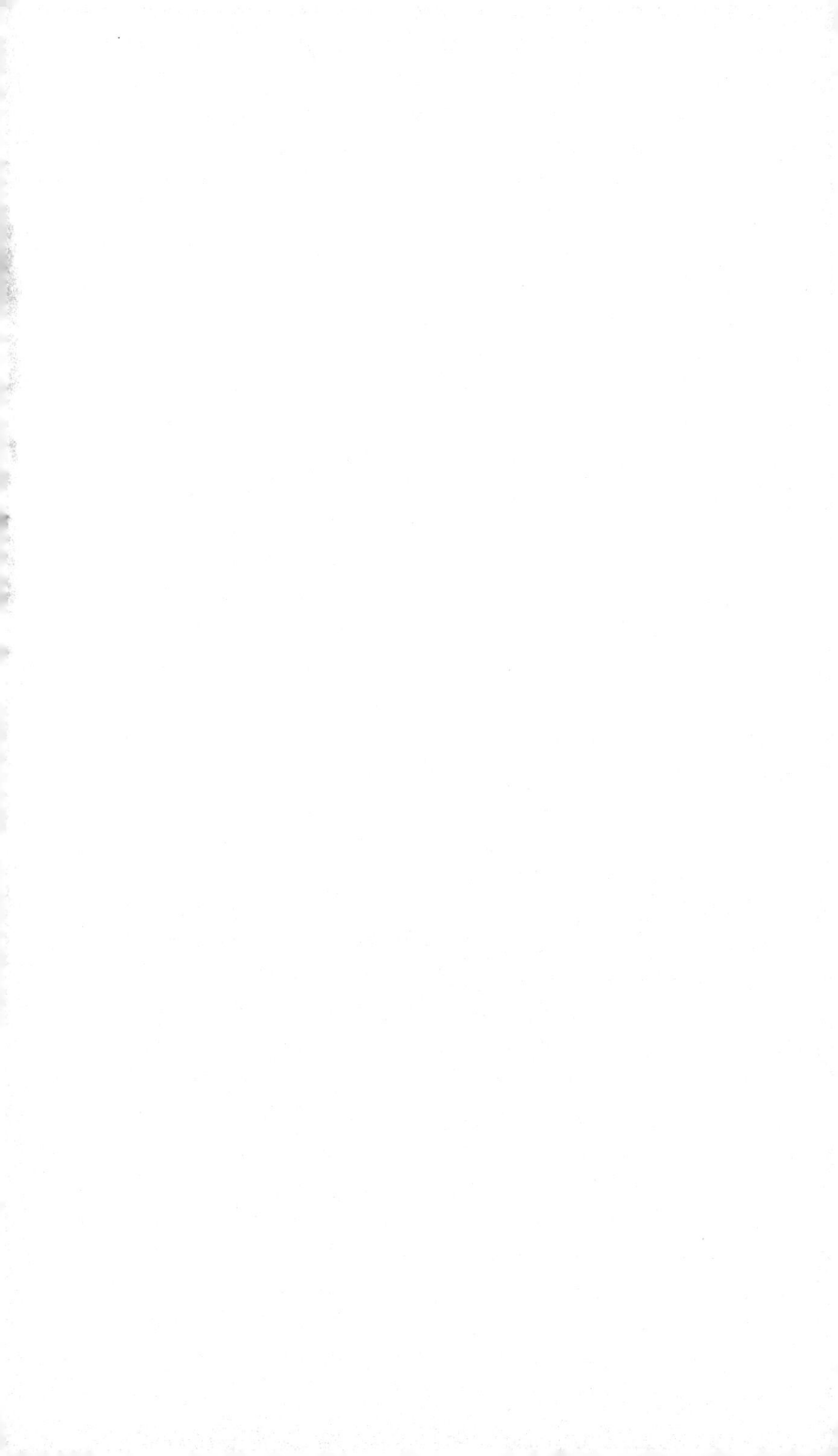